Gerard S. Doyle, M.D.

When There Is No Doctor ✚

Preventive and Emergency Home Healthcare in Challenging Times

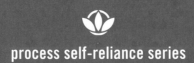

process self-reliance series

My thanks go to Jodi and Adam at Process/Feral House for their faith in an untried author and their support as I learned how to write a book. Gary, the editor, and Gregg's illustrations both made the book flow much better.

Above all, my undying love and gratitude go to my family. Thanks to Old Gringo for courageously demonstrating the most important lessons of this text. Our children have been our inspiration for so many things, including setting us on a path of trying to live more sustainably for them and their children. Most of all, my adoration belongs to Piper, my first editor and biggest booster! Her love and support have made everything possible.

—*Gerry Doyle*

....

This book is intended *solely* to stimulate discussion and learning. Some of the actions it describes may be illegal in your jurisdiction, while others are potentially dangerous. *You* have the responsibility to use this material wisely, safely and legally.

As you read this book, you will find specific diseases, therapies and treatments mentioned. The medical information provided in this book is, at best, of a general nature and cannot substitute for the advice of a qualified medical professional (for instance, a physician, veterinarian, nurse, or pharmacist, to name but a few). This book *must not* be construed as personal medical instruction or advice, and no action should be taken simply based on the contents of this volume.

The opinions and information contained in this book are believed to be accurate and sound, based on the best information available to the author, but readers who fail to consult appropriate health authorities assume the risk of *any* injuries or illness incurred from the use of this book. Medicine is a constantly growing and changing discipline, though, so the author and publisher cannot be held responsible for perceived errors or omissions.

When There Is No Doctor is part of the Process Self-Reliance Series

Process Media
1240 W. Sims Way Suite 124
Port Townsend, WA 98368
www.processmediainc.com

Cover design by Lissi Irwin
Interior Design by Bill Smith
Illustrations by Gregg Einhorn
ISBN 978-1-934170-11-3
Printed in the United States of America

Table of Contents

INTRODUCTION
Protecting and Restoring Health in Hard Times

IT IS A TYPICAL NIGHT IN THE EMERGENCY DEPARTMENT. THE WAITING ROOM IS FULL of patients, young and old, waiting to be seen by a doctor. Some of those waiting have family members there to help them while away the many hours before they can be seen. In many cases, those same family members are trying to succor the pain, to hold pressure on improvised dressings applied to wounds, or to get fluids down the throats of uncooperative, dehydrated children.

There is a strong odor of sweat and disease in the room. People not able to bathe or wash their clothing with soap for some time languish in their own filth. In addition to the stench, tension hangs in the air. Security presence is pointedly visible in hopes of keeping a lid on the simmering hostility the patients and their loved ones direct toward the staff.

Despite waiting a long time in these conditions for care, most patients are told by the nurses that there is nothing that can be done for them. Simple therapies like aspirin or Tylenol for fevers, or antacids for stomachaches are sometimes available. Patients moan in pain because of the severe shortages of narcotic pain medications and rationing of supplies in general. Those in need of treatment for more severe conditions may be admitted to the hospital, but the shortages of supplies and staff are just as acute on the inpatient wards. Diseases go undiagnosed and patients are left untreated.

The doctors at the hospital can only shrug and continue to write prescriptions they know pharmacists can't fill, as the medicine shortage is nationwide. Materials like surgical gloves and sutures are severely limited and many supplies once considered "disposable" need to be recycled for repeated use.

Some people are lucky because they can afford to go to clinics where their hard currency can be used to purchase needed supplies, and a few other clinics had the foresight to stockpile extra supplies in advance, but for the most part, few health care services are running at their previous levels.

Shortages of parts and energy have made ambulance services unavailable in most of the country, even the capital city, and have rendered tap water unsafe, forcing people to boil their water prior to drinking it. With garbage trucks idled, the trash sits uncollected on the streets for months.

Taken together, these changes have led to a decline in hygiene as well as serious setbacks in nutrition. Overall health suffers; infant mortality rates climb, and the death rate of the elderly increases by 20%. Fewer women choose to have babies due to poverty, but those who do are not spared, as maternal mortality almost doubles.

ALTHOUGH THIS NIGHTMARISH SCENARIO SEEMS FAR-FETCHED, IT ACTUALLY DID *happen*. This grim picture describes the so-called "special period" that occurred in Cuba in the 1990s following the collapse of the Soviet Union, on which Cuba was so dependent for material and economic as well as political support. Cubans responded with local action, growing food and medicinal plants in vacant lots and other urban areas, and health care workers reused and repurposed their supplies.

We must recognize that even under the best of circumstances, our system is as vulnerable as that of Cuba, or Argentina's during the 2002 economic crisis in that country.

More bluntly, as recipients of health care we are largely dependent on the hierarchy of medicine. Information that was once common knowledge has been obscured by the specialization inherent in modern, technologically intensive society. Previously, people were the ultimate generalist, able to largely provide the things they needed to survive for themselves, including health care. Although the self-care measures they applied may seem primitive, quaint and sometimes even dangerous now, knowledge had filtered down to a "man-on-the-street" level for many conditions and medical interventions.

Nowadays, medicine has become so specialized that not only are doctors unable to keep up with all areas of medicine, but their patients are also unfamiliar with many of these issues. These so-called "hidden hierarchies" can be deleterious to your ability to obtain good health advice if you're not proactive.

Despite the recent debate and onslaught of various bills that aim to bring wider access to health care (or insurance), the knowledge in this book will help you navigate life in a more healthy manner, helping you in your interactions with the health care system, your doctor, and other health care providers.

THIS IS A BOOK ABOUT SUSTAINABLE HEALTH, PRIMARILY HAVING TO DO WITH your health and *what you can do* to protect it, in bad times certainly, but also hopefully in good. I will narrow the focus to cover an unusual and perhaps provocative topic: how to help you ensure the health of those you love, yourself and, should you so choose, your community, when the world changes. *World* may come to mean your little town or the whole globe. It could change for a few days or weeks, or for a few years, or forever. It could change because of a flood, financial crisis, flu pandemic, or failure of our energy procurement, production or distribution systems.

I will not teach you to be a medical MacGyver, the lone survivalist who anticipates doing an appendectomy on himself or a loved one on the kitchen table with a steak knife and a few spoons, although I will discuss techniques of austere and improvised medicine for really hard times. My goal is to cover the crucial topics for preparedness and self-reliance when it comes to your health.

Maybe your ethics demand that you become aware of how to live a healthy lifestyle in a more ecologically conscious manner. Alternatively, you may want to know more about providing care beyond simple first aid, or how you can make lifestyle changes to improve your life despite the presence of a chronic disease. More importantly, I want to make you aware of and excited about the importance of sustainable health, and inform you about the resources available to help you start making the changes needed to move towards sustainability.

Regardless, after reading this, you will have a better understanding of how to plan and prepare for a variety of bad times, what disaster response planners call an "all hazards" approach to preparedness. My hopes in writing this are that you never have to use the information contained here. I hope that this information will be used to improve your baseline health so you can continue to lead a happy, long and productive life. In the event that the fecal matter hits the oscillating air circulator, I hope the mastery of the skills presented here, plus the planning done based on this information, will help you and your family make it through any rough times relatively unscathed. ●

CHAPTER 1

Our Situation

Where We Are, How We Got Here, Where We May Be Headed

YOU MAY HAVE HEARD TERMS LIKE "ENERGY DESCENT," "PETROCOLLAPSE" OR "PEAK OIL" used as shorthand for the societal changes expected to result from a decline in the supply of cheap, clean and easily accessible energy. Another term is *gridcrash*: the widespread disruption of modern life with its ease and convenience, either temporary or long-term.

The impending depletion of our fossil fuel-based energy supply is just one potential scenario. A crash could result from various causes: economic collapse, an outbreak of naturally occurring old or new diseases, war or terrorism, or the effects of climate change, just to mention a few forecast events. Every modern convenience could be impacted by each of these events, leading to what some call gridcrash. Modern medicine, as much as any sector of society, is highly dependent on an intact societal infrastructure. Infrastructure is composed of all the systems we count on in our modern, mobile, technology-dependent society: systems that produce and deliver our food, water, energy, clothing, building materials. These system—and thus our entire society—are dependent on a regular flow of fossil fuels (oil, coal, gas). Geologists and economists have been telling us for some time that these energy sources are running out.

Americans' dependence on modern medicine, which in turn is dependent on money, technology, and abundant oil, makes our health care system vulnerable to social, environmental and economic disruptions. We have already had glimpses of gridcrash, like when things happen as they did in Cuba in the '90s. Severe storms, earthquakes, and other natural disasters can debilitate energy and transportation systems, resulting in bridge collapses, blackouts and other disruptions.

Throughout history, health has been produced primarily by improvements in societal infrastructure. In turn, these improvements are made possible by two distinctly non-medical factors: economic growth and cheap, reliable energy sources. A map of which societies have produced most medical "breakthroughs" looks a lot like a map of who has the highest GNP or who is producing and consuming the most energy.

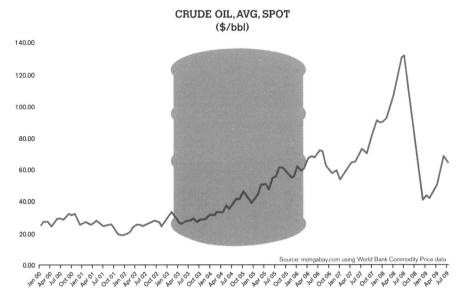

CRUDE OIL, AVG, SPOT
($/bbl)

Source: mongabay.com using World Bank Commodity Price data

Petroleum-based supplies are the rule in modern medicine.

No sector of society is more dependent on cheap energy than health care. Like much of modern life, health care today is technologically amazing, but that reliance on technology cuts both ways. Petroleum-based synthetic medicines and supplies must be manufactured and shipped, patients and staff moved, buildings lighted and temperatures controlled, food procured and prepared, laundry washed and dried, and computers and diagnostic and therapeutic equipment powered and maintained in any modern hospital.

AS OIL SUPPLIES DECLINE, PRICES WILL RISE, AND ALL OF THESE ACTIVITIES WILL BECOME more expensive. We have seen how increasing oil prices have an effect on the price and availability of food, and just about everything else. We are forced to admit that the Internet is not the only tangled web we have woven.

Again, this is not a new problem: the OPEC oil embargo in the mid-1970s led to recognition of the critical reliance of society (and the health care "system" especially) on oil. Forward-looking authors asked how long we would continue to have access to the resources that allow us to have good health care. Although not expressed as succinctly, they recognized the need to encourage the relatively profligate health care system to "reduce, reuse and recycle."

Despite these connections, no such efforts were undertaken. Health care, like much of society at large, patches its major problems and moves on without

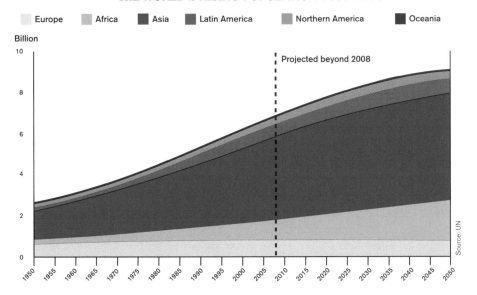

THE WORLD'S RISING POPULATION 1950–2050

Europe   Africa   Asia   Latin America   Northern America   Oceania

Billion

Projected beyond 2008

Source: UN

system-wide efforts to eliminate the underlying weaknesses often at fault. At the present time it appears that very few people in health care are examining these issues openly. The modern health care system in America is not united or organized for unified action, so there is little coordinated preparation for a gridcrash scenario, and peak oil and the economic changes it will bring about have gotten even less attention.

While these potential problems are intrinsic to the US health care system we have today, there are other external threats. The health care system is currently constructed as a business, and like a lot of business, medicine relies on modern management techniques to control costs. Hospitals use "just in time" stocking of supplies, often made overseas due to lower manufacturing costs. Few supplies are kept on hand for a "rainy day." Staffing in health care today is "casual." meaning nurses and many other staff members work 2-3 part-time jobs rather than having loyalty to any single employer. The health care system is running near capacity and is a fragmented group of competitors, rather than a cohesive unit. Even public agencies like county hospitals and local health departments are "stovepiped" and have to work hard to coordinate plans with other organizations within the same governmental body.

Society to a large extent has also fallen into a business model driven largely by pharmaceutical companies and tertiary care centers. Primary care and prevention, which ideally would form the bulwark of our health care system, are downplayed. Rescue measures abound, but cost much more than prevention. So-called "lifestyle diseases" (because they may be prevented or treatable early on if addressed by lifestyle modification) are instead treated with pills and surgery. Even Hollywood has noticed: There aren't many shows about the noble family practitioner discussing smoking cessation, but we have *ER*; the show *Biggest Loser* is a hit, but not many viewers work out while tuned in to the Fitness Channel in hopes of avoiding recruitment for *Biggest Loser*.

All of these factors make health care vulnerable to gridcrash. Current estimates are that in the event of a moderate to severe influenza pandemic (as happened in 1918, 1957 and most recently 1968), between 30 and 40% of the workforce will not show up for work for 6 to 8 weeks. Think about how this could ripple through society: the producers, shippers, stockers and retailers, all short of staff. How will that affect our ability to get our prescription or over-the-counter medications?

Imagine a "bird flu" or H5N1 avian influenza outbreak in Asia, with its current 60% mortality rate. Consider that about 80% of disposable health care supplies used in this country come from Asia. Only 13% of generic drugs submitted for FDA approval two years ago were made in the US; six times as many were made in Asia. Do you see any potential problems here?

Any of these events could jeopardize the smooth functioning of our current health care structure, but what would happen if other systems were to be affected simultaneously? Some "peak oil" proponents predict that we will be growing our own food, making our own clothes, struggling to light and heat (or cool) our homes and disposing of our own wastes. All of these activities could put us at risk for illness and injury. These risks would be on top of the burden from lifestyle diseases so prevalent today like diabetes, obesity and hypertension. Our health could be jeopardized when the infrastructure is "down" even only for a few weeks, even if the health care system recovers eventually.

While some consumers of fuel and food have reacted by adopting "sustainability" measures like riding mass transit or using human powered transport, retrofitting their homes with solar panels, or eating locally grown foods, there has been no consumer-initiated, market-driven response to the vulnerability of the health care system to gridcrash. This book seeks to start filling that void.

Most folks look at sustainability as a way of living with minimal impact on the planet and its health, or reliance on its resources. Others, anticipating gridcrash scenarios, see it as a way of living in such a way that their lives will, at worst, be minimally impacted by the occurrence of such a scenario.

Sustainable health looks at both of these as inseparable issues. By living a sustainable life now your health will likely be better and more sustainable. You will reduce the impact of your own health on the planet and its people, and in return, there will be less impact on your health if things get really bad. The planning and preparation you do in advance will make your health less likely to suffer under any circumstance. The goal is for you to become more self-reliant, and less dependent on technology and nonrenewable sources of energy.

Paranoia! some say. These things will never happen. We will have newer technologies that will give us renewable, clean energy. There will be no more devastating depressions, world wars or large-scale terrorist attacks. Modern medicine can quickly come up with vaccines and therapies for future epidemics. Besides, how long have they warned us about the bird flu? Where has it been?

Even if there is no big crash, being able to provide basic health care interventions for yourself, or for friends and family simply makes sense. If you travel, especially to under-developed nations, or if you engage in outdoor activities, especially in remote areas, the simple hygiene and first aid measures discussed here can be lifesaving. This is especially true given that deaths in these settings are most often due to injury and heart disease, while infections like traveler's diarrhea make many more people sick, even during adventures in the developed world.

Staying at home may not guarantee your total safety and comfort, as we have learned from countless minor "disasters" like storms, floods, strikes and power outages. Hurricanes like Katrina, floods, fires and winter storms all may render infrastructure in your small part of the world nonfunctional for a period of time. Being able to meet basic health needs in such times is essential.

If you are planning to any extent on having easy access to health care, whether it be doctor visits, prescription or over-the-counter medications, or other accoutrements of modern health care, you should anticipate what you would need to do for yourself or your loved ones to remain healthy in the event of short or long-term disaster. Do you know enough about your own condition to allow you to make good lifestyle choices in terms of diet and activity as well as non-pharmacologic therapies for your disease? Are there other alternatives such as herbs you could use in an emergency situation? The time to find out is now, and not after you've learned that the doctor's office is closed, the pharmacy is out of the medication you need and the hospital will only see patients who have flu symptoms.

Where We Should Be Going

SUSTAINABILITY, LIKE GRIDCRASH AND ITS SYNONYMS, IS A TERM IN VOGUE LATELY. IN OUR modern, energy-dependent, technology-intensive society, our daily needs are met through a variety of mechanisms. This sustainability is shaped like a pyramid: A lot of what is essential for sustaining life is the base, while other

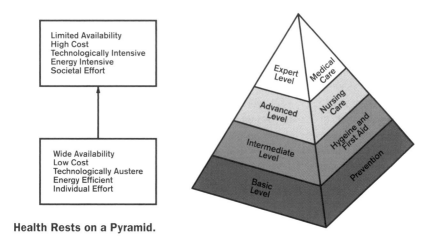

Health Rests on a Pyramid.

conveniences take place higher up. To "climb" or move up the pyramid takes some combination of training, energy, technology and societal support.

As an example, we can meet some transportation needs ourselves: going out to get the mail, walking down the block to the neighborhood store or around the corner to the local elementary school. We rely on technology and energy as well as specialized training and the infrastructure of our society to drive to the mall and, even more so, in order to fly across the country to visit grandma.

Our health and medical care both rest on similar pyramids. The base needs are relatively simple and don't demand a lot of infrastructure. We must be able to build the base of the pyramid ourselves. We should be able to climb at least part-way up ourselves as well, just in case the energy, technology and society aren't there to the degree that they are now to provide the care found further up the pyramid. Luckily, the base of the health care sustainability pyramid is easily accessible.

In our world today, many of the skills and knowledge for functions low down on the pyramids of meeting our daily needs have been taken from us by the division of labor and the "need" for convenience. We rely on "public health" workers to provide a lot of the preventive services we need to help ensure our health, just as we rely on the medical infrastructure to rescue us from diseases borne of our folly or our fate.

In the same way that we may need to take over the very basics of some food production (our own backyard garden?) or transportation (riding a bike to work or walking?) in the event of a gridcrash, so we must be able to take over some of the health care needs currently met by our medical system through its use of training, energy, technology and society. This book aims to help you to shore up your health care pyramid's base and to learn how to make your way up the health care sustainability pyramid.

In this book I will try to make you an expert in health care for times when there is *no* doctor, but with a bit of a twist: I believe that an expert is someone who does *the basics* very well. In this model, the basics are naturally those things that form the base of the pyramid. These are activities best mastered before gridcrash, indeed before even a brief infrastructure disruption occurs. Daily use of these basics after you master them could also improve your life right now.

You should focus on preparing body, mind and spirit for these presaged trying times. Plan so that you and your home, your family and your neighborhood are ready. Only after that should you focus on the actual medical care aspects of health after gridcrash.

Prevention and public health will be the key basics. If you keep your living environment clean, limit the potential for spread of infections from person to person and animal to person, keep fit to maximize your health and minimize chronic disease, and practice sensible injury control, you have gone a long way to being an expert in sustainable health.

Next up the pyramid are simple "first aid" and supportive nursing-care interventions that most of us have learned by watching them done to us over the years. Since ancient times, and until only very recently, most physicians would admit that most of what they did was gently nudge nature in the right direction and let her take her course, as most of the time we can heal ourselves. In many cases, we just need the balance tipped in our favor: getting extra rest and fluids to fight off a cold, icing a sprain to limit pain and inflammation, keeping a cut clean and dry to prevent infection and speed healing, exercising to foster rehabilitation from an injury, and the like. When you finish with this book, I hope you will be on the path to being an expert in these things, and you will also know how to learn more.

If that is still not enough, I will cover how to help when things really get bad, the so-called "the end of the world as we know it" scenario. We will cover some common symptoms or injuries and how to deal with them in the event of truly catastrophic events. Maybe you want to know how prisoners performed surgery under anesthesia while living in jungle huts and wearing loincloths under conditions of brutal deprivation. Perhaps you just are curious if honey can really be used as a medicine.

A lot of this info will be things we learned in the past but have forgotten as we relied on cheap energy and technology to help us make our way up the health sustainability pyramid. Some will be improvised medicine learned in austere settings like indigenous societies and people ravaged by poverty and war, as well as those in prisons and POW camps and at sea. Here, too, I will try to point out ways for you to learn more about this stuff.

I would not recommend that you plan to do things outside your comfort zone: I don't mean you should be able to do surgery in a tent, unless you want to *and* are willing to do what it takes to be able to do it safely and well. You should seek to find a level of training, and ideally experience, needed to manage conditions that you can reasonably expect to encounter in foreseeable scenarios. I will give you some resources, Internet and book-based, that will allow you to work on these issues yourself.

Just as a single household in a large city could not expect to meet all its need for food nor fight off roving gangs of marauders all by itself, you are probably not in a position to be able to provide all the health care you will need by yourself. There is a lot of talk these days about "community sustainability." This is the idea of a neighborhood or village coming together as an *intentional community* and sharing assets: skills, tools and supplies. Together, the whole will be much more than the sum of its parts. In the same way, you should know your family, friends and neighbors. Then, be ready and able to team with them to make your little village self-sustaining.

I won't tell you how to care for many specific conditions, injuries or diseases. I do encourage you to use the resources I will give to find the training you desire that fits within your lifestyle (time, money, family and level of concern about the future).

As part of any preparation, you must not only prepare your mind but also be ready bodily and spiritually. No serious discussion of gridcrash can take place without acknowledging that physical and emotional stresses will be on the rise; as with any preparedness activity it makes sense to prepare for these stresses in advance, not to try to cram in measures in a panic as disaster is looming or once it strikes.

To that end, I will describe functional fitness and how to gain it in preparation for having to rely more upon your body, in the same way our forebears did. In addition, I will give you some tools for safeguarding your spirit (your emotional health) that have been used by others in very trying circumstances. This information could be the most important as we will see from examples where people didn't have those tools.

What about supplies? Aren't they as important as this mind-body-spirit tripe? Many survival books and survivalist blogs publish lists of first aid supplies that would rival a small clinic, even including some surgical supplies. This is putting the cart before the horse.

Everything you do in terms of "stocking up" must flow from your ability to use the tools at hand. Unlike woodworking or gardening and many other preparedness activities, in medicine there is little opportunity to practice skills and techniques on live subjects, so having a kick-ass medical kit without the skills and knowledge to use it is poor planning. Poor planning is tantamount to planning a poor outcome.

More importantly, you *must* be able to prevent most illnesses and injuries under any circumstances: Prevention is worth a pound of cure, and this is essential when that pound of cure may cost too much time, energy, money or pain, or may not even be available. Because of this, the focus will initially be on hygiene, fitness, and the like to avoid the need to rescue yourself or loved ones with improvised, less-than-ideal medical care. If you do the basics well, you will be an expert, even if you cannot perform surgery in a tent.

Having said all of this, I hope to be able to impart to you some ideas on useful planning and preparation. In addition, there will be small vignettes throughout the coming chapters—tips on how to make due when things are very bad. See *Honey As Medicine?* for an example of one of these vignettes.

Honey as Medicine? TIP

HONEY HAS BEEN A "STANDARD" MEDICAL TREATMENT SINCE ANCIENT TIMES.

Civilizations from China to Egypt, Greece and Rome used the golden nectar for treatment of wounds as well as diseases of the gastrointestinal tract. Both the Bible and the Koran mention it, most famously perhaps in the idea of a "land flowing with milk and honey."

Since then, newer synthetic medications have supplanted honey's traditional roles within modern medicine. Despite this, many cultures in Africa, Asia, Oceana and the Americas continue to use honey.

What's more, honey is making a comeback in Western medicine. Recent clinical trials show that honey has beneficial effects in treating cough in children, burns and other wounds, and gastrointestinal infections. Many of these effects are due to *hygroscopic* nature of honey. This describes a key property caused by the high concentration of sugars in the syrupy liquid: Honey sucks the water out of bacteria and fungi to keep them from growing. This action also helps minimize swelling of injured tissues, speeding healing of wounds. Finally, enzymes in the honey seem to have directly toxic effects on the bugs, including generation of hydrogen peroxide.

Honeys from different plant and bee combinations vary in terms of their antibacterial activity, but some have been shown to suppress growth of "*superbugs*" like Pseudomonas and MRSA that are very problematic for patients with complicated wounds.

In 2007, some pediatricians did a study where they looked at the "Effect of Honey, Dextromethorphan, and No Treatment on Nocturnal Cough and Sleep Quality for Coughing Children and Their Parents." The findings suggested that kids who are given a bedtime dose of buckwheat honey do a bit better in terms of their nighttime cough and difficulty sleeping than those who got a dose of Dextromethorphan (the active ingredient in many over-the-counter cough suppressants). They did significantly better than those children given a placebo.

The dark "buckwheat" honey used in this study can be dosed like this: Age 2 to 5, ½ teaspoon; Age 6 to 11, 1 teaspoon; Age 12-18, 2 teaspoons. Honey is NOT recommended for children under 1 year of age (due to the risk of infant botulism as discussed below).

Honey has also been shown to help shorten the course of diarrhea in cases of bacterial dysentery in the developing world. Honey can be used as a 5% solution (about 1 teaspoonful in 4 ounces total) instead of sugar in homemade oral rehydration therapy fluid. (See *Tip: Fluid Administration Without an IV*)

NOTE

Honey for use in wound care is more complicated, primarily due to the issue of botulism. The spores for the bacteria that cause botulism can sometimes be harbored in honey sold as food. This can cause infantile botulism if children less than a year old eat honey. There is some concern that honey placed on wounds, especially deep or dirty wounds, will find favorable conditions to cause botulism within the wounds. Because of this, many producers of medical honey sterilize it with gamma radiation. Of course this kind of medical honey is less likely to be available after a bad gridcrash event.

Others, particularly in the developing world, have used honey from the hive without reporting any of these problems. In these settings, honey is used to saturate a dressing that is then placed on the wound or burn.

Apitherapy, the use of bee products like honey or propolis (a waxy glue-like material found holding hives together) is already popular in Europe as well as Australia and New Zealand. Future research may lead to many other medical uses for bees that could help take the sting out of gridcrash health.

FINALLY, I WANT TO SAY A FEW WORDS ABOUT SOME PHILOSOPHICAL STUFF. THIS IS A BOOK for the "peak geek." the doomsayer who knows that a gridcrash may happen, while again it may not, but who recognizes that it is better to have prepared for the worst, as these preparations help even if the stuff doesn't hit the fan. An all-hazards approach can make you more prepared for a short, small scale disaster or a long emergency with a gradual decline in the standard of living. Some of these measures make sense in a time of economic austerity, too, by making you more self-sufficient and thereby potentially saving you some money. In the end, though, we have to get ready for the world that can reasonably be foreseen, not the world as we *wish* it to be.

In this regard, you must determine for yourself if you wish to be in denial (the fact that this book is in your hands makes that outcome unlikely), if you want to spend your time working to prevent gridcrash or if you want to get ready for it. Do you want to invest effort and time into convincing a few of your fellow citizens to take some steps to prevent gridcrash, or directing your limited resources to making yourself, your family and your community ready (which offers some respite to the ecosystem). I am in the latter camp, and suspect you may be, too.

Either way, it all begins with you: denial, activism or preparation. Failing to decide upon any one of these does not eliminate the need for a decision. ●

CHAPTER 2

Preparation

Make Your Body Ready

IN ORDER TO MAXIMIZE YOUR CHANCES OF COMING THROUGH ANY GRIDCRASH SCENARIO, YOU must optimize your health before any event that might significantly disrupt societal infrastructure. This requires that you begin to aggressively protect your health *now*, including maximizing your fitness and minimizing your risk for illness and injury. Part of this can be done through simple lifestyle choices and, as is so often the case in life, we *know* what we should do but don't always *do* what we know we should.

Before gridcrash, fitness is a highly desirable trait: A *New England Journal of Medicine* study showed that for each hour you spend engaged in vigorous exercise, you are rewarded with an additional two hours of life, probably of a higher quality.

After any societal cataclysm, a good level of fitness will be more than just a way to improve your quality of life or looks, or to extend your years on this Earth. Fitness will be essential to survival. The fight for survival will be just that at times: a physical struggle. You must be fit for that struggle. This gives new meaning to "survival of the fittest."

Physical fitness, like money, is fungible: Once made, it can be spent in a variety of manners. What does this mean? Fitness gained from riding your bike to work may help improve your ability to walk to the store, grow crops in the garden, chop firewood, push a wheelbarrow up a hill or run from danger. If you are fit and healthy, you can expect that these tasks will be much easier for you than for somebody else who has not done any regular exercise.

A good base of fitness will keep your weight down, enhance your ability to recover from physical insults and emotional stresses, and improve your tolerance to extremes of weather such as heat waves. In all likelihood you will also have larger mental reserves, making it easier to think clearly under stressful situations or when you are tired. The endorphins released during vigorous exercise also improve your mental outlook in general and improve your morale in hard times, making depression and anxiety less likely.

Functional Fitness for a Crash

IF YOU ARE READING THIS, YOU ARE PROBABLY ACTIVELY ENGAGED IN SOME FORM OF A FIT-ness regimen already. It is much less likely that you are someone who smokes, eats to excess, binge-drinks alcohol or plays video games at the expense of even a modicum of exercise. Still, this chapter is important: Hard times call for hard folks. Not necessarily emotionally hard, but people who are able to meet the potential physical demands of a world without modern conveniences.

How should you go about getting fit? While treadmills, rowing machines, elliptical trainers, yoga and group exercise classes are all beneficial for developing some elements of fitness, and may even be fun, I would argue that you need more than this–or if not more, perhaps a different approach. I like to call it *functional fitness*.

Functional fitness is just what it says: fitness that allows you to perform functions, not just the contrived motions of the elliptical trainer or aerobics class. Functional means you can *DO* something useful. In the variety of scenarios following gridcrash, these functions are things that allow you to get done the things you need to do in order to eat and drink, have shelter, travel and the like. Again, these are things we take for granted today, but may not be able to so easily in the future. I mean the strength and endurance to collect firewood, dig a latrine, walk several miles to the store and carry back a load of groceries and to complete other similar tasks.

How do I suggest you go about obtaining this functional fitness? Well, after you have a base of fitness from the gym or your recreational pursuits, you should start doing those activities that you may end up being *forced* to do by circumstances. This offers you some distinct advantages. First, you can get in a good workout. Fitness is also somewhat specific: We are what we train to become. Doing diverse tasks will build muscle strength and agility over the whole body. As your agility for these tasks improves, you will be less prone to mistakes that can lead to injury, especially as you learn new tasks. Finally, there are time and potential money savings realized by combining your workout with sustainability measures.

For example, let's say you have a wood stove in your home. Instead of paying someone to deliver wood to your house already cut and split, do the following: Put on boots and grab a pack. Go to a wooded area near your house (with permission or permits as required). Bring a saw and a splitting maul, plus protective equipment. Find trees that have been blown over and section them with the saw, then split them. Carry a load out to your car or truck. Repeat. Not only will you now have firewood, but you will have learned some useful skills and improved your functional fitness level.

Think about what tasks you might need to do to keep your family or your home going after gridcrash. Heat from that woodstove may be lifesaving, but only if YOU can get the fuel. Veggies and starches from the garden? Can you grow them? Not "harvest" them from the store, but turn the compost pile, hoe the row for the seeds, bend and pull weeds, and all the other tasks needed to be self-sufficient, day in and day out? Maybe you just need to get a few miles to work; what if you have to walk or bicycle because there's no gas and the buses sit idle?

These questions are important because if you are not healthy and in good shape before bad times, you probably WON'T be able to get healthy and fit afterward. The time to prepare is now; waiting until you "need to prepare" might be too late. It is best to figure out NOW if you have a problem and then fix it—be it a shoulder that won't let you split wood with a maul, a knee that keeps you from carrying a load of groceries home or a back that limits you to two hours of gardening per day.

But you say you can run a marathon. Good for you. You have a great fitness base. Maybe instead of running 5-6 days per week, you should diversify and do some functional fitness activities—walking or bicycling to the store or other brief errands, or working in the garden. As in nature, diversity builds resilience. Repetition is important too, so choosing activities that you enjoy doing will help you sustain your exercise regime. What about swimming, rock climbing, rowing, cross country skiing? At least do something that covers all of the major components of fitness—strength, speed, endurance, agility, and flexibility. Make sure you don't neglect major muscle groups or motions.

Maybe you live in the city, and the idea of playing Paul Bunyan is impractical. If so, look for ideas like "boot camp." "strongman" or "dinosaur training" style workouts. These old-school training philosophies focus more on functional fitness attributes that aren't usually emphasized in gyms.

I think that, in our modern world, we have several glaring weaknesses when it comes to attaining functional fitness. First is load carrying. Look at folks from the rest of the world: Huge numbers of people in Africa, Asia and Central and South America have to carry food, water or fuel many miles. Forget about walking unladen; they have that down, too. In my mind, you need to be able to cover at least 4 miles with 30-40 pounds on your back in an hour. Unsupported: no stops, no food, no water. We evolved as bipeds, so this is programmed into our biology. Start by walking one mile at a brisk pace, then add a little weight, gradually increasing your pace, distance, and weight.

There is a reason most elite military units use long marches under heavy packs as part of their training and selection processes. The fatigue they induce brings out our personalities. As Vince Lombardi said, "Fatigue makes cowards of us all." A benefit of this kind of work is learning how you respond to stress,

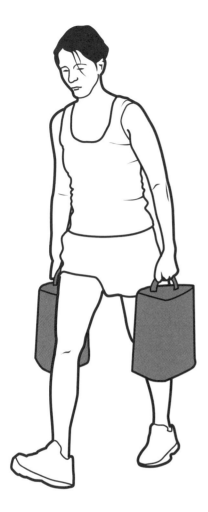

"Farmer's walk"

both bodily and more importantly emotionally. Believe me when I tell you that even if you have a stressful life now, it will be worse after the lights have been off for a week!

Another deficient area for a lot of people is grip strength. Many of us have soft hands from our relatively pampered lives, and weak grips result from a lifestyle that doesn't force us to use our hands. Even fit people don't do a lot of exercises that force them to use their grip. What happens when you need to carry a five-gallon bucket of water, waste or food, repetitively or over long distance? How about swinging an axe or a maul or a sledge to clear land or split firewood?

Finally, many of us are fair-weather exercisers: If the weather isn't PERFECT, we head indoors for the workout, the iPod in our ears, the TV in our face, and the water bottle close at hand. A gridcrash scenario will force you to bear the summer day's heat and humidity, and the winter night's cold and dark. Now is the time to get used to them, too.

There are lots of potential gym exercises suggested to help remedy these weak areas, but as Nike's famous slogan says: "Just Do It"! Do those things that maybe modern life and our neighbors discourage us from doing. Ditch the snow blower and shovel the driveway and walkways. Walk or bike to work or the store. Put on a backpack and go hiking on the weekend instead of playing golf or lounging by a pool.

If you have to rely on a gym, there are alternatives. While many personal trainers in trendy health clubs with lots of chrome dumbbells can be heard exhorting their clients to build core strength, you will go a long way toward this kind of fitness with simple body weight exercises like pull-ups, push-ups and sit-ups. Add "Farmer's walk" where you simply carry a dumbbell (or similar weight) in each hand and walk as far as you can. You get both grip strength and load carrying benefits at the same time.

If you don't want to do this, you could walk around your back yard carrying a 5 Gallon bucket in each hand; simply add water as your strength and endurance improve. Similarly, you could carry groceries from the store or books from the library in a pack, walking each way. Could there be a simpler way to functional fitness?

Healthy Habits Before Gridcrash

BODY PREPARATION ALSO INCLUDES MAXIMIZING YOUR HEALTH. LET'S SAY THAT YOU ENJOY more than the occasional drink, or maybe you smoke a few cigarettes with coworkers each day, but you say you "can kick the habit" anytime. I have only two words for you: Quit now! Not only are these habits a drag on your health, but after the widespread disruption caused by gridcrash, you may be forced to go "cold turkey".

Do you know how you will be affected when this happens? If you really can't quit that easily, are you willing to incur the added cost of these items, which is certain to rise in the future? This concern goes even for folks like me that rely on that morning cuppa Joe to get us going. Ever had a caffeine withdrawal headache? The time to find these things out is now, not later when you are stressed because your stocks just tanked, or there is an hourlong line to buy rationed gas or a curfew because of a recent terrorist attack. Try a "drug holiday" where you see what happens when you quit, cold turkey, even for a day.

If you have more of a problem, either with frequent heavy use of alcohol, routine use prescription medications like pain pills or sedatives, or if you use illegal drugs, you are probably not reading this book. Still, if use of alcohol or drugs is an issue for you or a loved one, keep in mind that withdrawal from them can not only be painful, but could kill you in some cases. Again, the time is now to do something about this.

Most of the determinants of health that we can affect ourselves are related to our lifestyle habits: diet, exercise, rest, vices and the like. Genetics impact our health, as do the nature of our fallible biological structures, but we can do very little to change the impact of these on our health. Much as we are what we eat, we are also what we drink, smoke or otherwise put in our bodies. We are what we *are* because of what we *do* to ourselves.

A recurring theme of this book is that now is the time to prepare, while things are relatively good. If the predictions of climate change, economic despair or petrocollapse come true it will be even harder than it is now to use willpower to bring about positive changes, be it in your habits or in any other area of preparation addressed in this book.

Nutritional Optimization of Health Prior to a Crash

DIET AND NUTRITION HAVE ALWAYS BEEN CONTROVERSIAL AREAS. YOU CAN FIND PASSIONATE advocates for just about any kind of diet: The low-carb, high-fat fans decry the high-carb, low-fat proponents. Some say megadose vitamins are necessary and could prevent cancer, while others say well-balanced diets are just fine without supplements. Other folks have come up with even more exotic or exacting, or both, dietary advise. Look in any bookstore, and you will find a huge array of diet books. The grizzled sages among us say that if any single diet worked we wouldn't need all these books! Still, now is the time to find a healthy diet that you can follow. I can't pick one for you, so it's up to you to find out how to have a nutritionally sound diet.

From my viewpoint, working towards self-sufficiency dictates that you learn about diet and then make choices you feel are best for yourself and your family. Having said that, your doctor or a health educator or nutritionist, if you have access to one through your insurance or your job, can steer you in the right direction. In addition, the USDA and a number of other organizations have published some basic guidelines on what constitutes good nutrition.

For all intents and purposes, the key to sound nutrition is probably variety and moderation in everything. There should be a focus on "whole foods" with as much of your diet being fresh foods like fruits and vegetables as possible, with a minimum of pre-packaged processed foods. You should especially avoid foods high in simple sugars, fats or preservatives. See the list of resources at the end of the chapter for ideas on how to optimize your nutrition.

We have already looked at the medicinal use of one food, honey. There are a number of other foods that have also been shown to have useful clinical effects. This has been known since the days of Hippocrates, the founder of the western medical tradition, who said "Let food be thy medicine."

Sticking with that theme, we know that diets rich in fruits and vegetables help reduce the risk of cancer, while processed foods and meats are associated with heightened cancer risks. In general, a diet composed of whole foods like fresh fruits and vegetables but low in processed foods with their simple sugars and unhealthy fats is best overall. Some foods, though, seem to possess additional benefits.

Medicinal foods offer benefits in that they are likely to be cheaper than a lot of medicines and may have fewer side effects, plus you can grow your own, and they are dual-use—you may get a yummy meal with your medicine, a different take on Julie Andrews' spoonful of sugar!

Teas are consumed world wide because they are pleasant, socially acceptable, economical, and safe. Teas contain biologically active compounds that may prevent a wide variety of diseases: It is the best source of an antioxidant class called *flavonoids*, and contains many other useful components such as vitamins and fluoride. Based on this, doctors have identified many potential beneficial medical and health effects of a number of teas, which are under study for further uses even now.

Black tea has been shown to generally give a positive effect on health. Evidence has shown risk reduction for coronary artery disease at intakes of at least 3 cups per day, and for improved antioxidant status at intakes of 1 to 6 cups per day.

Green tea may also help to reduce the risk of cardiovascular disease and some forms of cancer. It also promotes oral health and may have anti-hypertensive effects, help to control body weight, protect against solar ultraviolet radiation, and increase bone mineral density.

Extensive use of spices probably came about when folks recognized that not only did they add flavor to foods but they seemed to offer some preservative effects, making foods last longer in the time before refrigeration. These benefits probably derived from either anti-microbial or anti-oxidant effects, and it is these effects that earn spices the focus of modern medicine in the search for new drugs from old herbs.

Garlic has been used as a medicinal agent for thousands of years, starting with the ancient Egyptians. In more modern times, Louis Pasteur, considered the father of infectious disease, reported the antibacterial effects of garlic in the 1850s. Garlic seems to have other immune system boosting effects as well.

Garlic is currently recommended as an aid to lowering cholesterol, reducing other cardiovascular risk factors, and for anti-neoplastic (cancer fighting) and antimicrobial properties. For these effects, you need about 1-2 raw garlic cloves per day, which some feel can lead to unpleasant breath and body odors as well as gas and stomach upset; topical use can lead to burns and dermatitis.

Some studies have shown about 10% reduction in cholesterol in those taking a garlic supplement compared to those taking a placebo. There is an ongoing clinical trial to characterize the usefulness of garlic, sponsored and funded by the US Government through the National Center for Complementary and Alternative Medicine (NCCAM).

There is weak evidence that garlic improves blood pressure, lowers blood sugar in diabetics, reduces the stickiness of blood platelets (the effect we seek in prescribing aspirin for heart attacks) and slows development of atherosclerosis.

Taken together, these effects if real could not only make garlicky foods taste good but reduce the rate of heart attack and stroke, two of the biggest killers of the modern age.

In terms of cancer, folks who eat a lot of garlic and similar vegetables (allium class like onions) show lower occurrence of stomach and colon cancer than those who consume lower amounts of these foods.

Garlic extracts exert activity against bacteria, viruses and fungi *in vitro* ("in glass" or test-tube based experiments). Currently there seems to be very little clinical evidence of useful antimicrobial effects, but garlic has traditionally been used for a wide range of infectious conditions.

Ginger works to help reduce the severity of symptoms from osteoarthritis, the degenerative form that occurs from wear and tear associated with age, overuse and prior injury. It has been shown to work, although not as well as ibuprofen, in relieving knee pain; presumably it would help pain in other joints as well.

The NCCAM has evaluated the available studies, and has also funded investigators to study interactions of ginger with some drugs (immunosuppressants), plus its effect of reducing nausea in patients receiving chemotherapy, and the safety and effectiveness of its use for preventive health purposes, as well as its impact on inflammation. When these studies are done, ginger's utility will be clearly outlined and available for incorporation into mainstream therapy, and also for post-gridcrash use. Ginger may not be a true "universal remedy" as some label it now, but it may be proven in the future to have widespread medicinal value.

Another spice that can help with inflammatory diseases like arthritis is curcumin, a major constituent of the spice turmeric. This staple of Ayurvedic medicine seems very safe as a topical or oral treatment of pain from arthritis.

Many other foods have utility as either preventive measures or as therapeutic agents:

Vitamin D (the sunshine vitamin) seems to improve respiratory health, and may reduce the impact of tuberculosis, respiratory viruses and asthma and emphysema. Supplements also have been shown to increase lifespan.

Essential fatty acids like omega-3 and omega-6 fatty acids (that our bodies can't make) from fish oils, berries, nuts and eggs have a wide range of benefits, including reducing cardiovascular diseases, depression and dementia, among other maladies.

Probiotics (helpful living organisms found in foods like yogurt, sourdough, sauerkraut) help maintain intestinal health and seem to play a role in protecting us from a variety of inflammatory reactions that could cause us problems ranging from irritable bowel syndrome to preterm labor and hospital-borne infections.

Cloves, oregano, cinnamon, pepper, ginger and garlic have high levels of antioxidants that may protect against cancer and vascular disease.

A wide variety of edible mushrooms seem to have anti-tumor activity in lab studies, though none have been proven to treat or prevent cancer.

It also pays to remember that obesity– and the diabetes and other metabolic changes that come with it– can impair immunity and put you at risk for infections, so go easy on the food.

Functional foods, those like those discussed above, may offer the utility of medicines while having advantages like ease of procurement or cultivation. Some may have fewer side effects than drugs used to treat the same condition, although no medicine, even natural, is truly free of side effects for every user. Still, keep an eye on sites like those listed in the appendix for further word on the value of these low-tech dual-use commodities.

Water is a key nutrient that most people ignore. Humans are about 70% water. Most of us probably don't drink enough water; we know that some physical and mental performance measures are worsened by dehydration, beyond simply feeling worse. A 2-3% drop in body water makes you less attentive to details and you will have to concentrate more and work harder on simple tasks. More importantly, though, is that folks who are dehydrated feel worse: They feel more tired and less alert. Any parent knows that kids get confused, irritable and lethargic when they're thirsty.

In addition, people frequently confuse hunger and thirst. Try it yourself: When you feel hungry, drink 8 ounces of water and wait. See if the hunger passes or persists before you chow down!

Staying well-hydrated helps to prevent dental disease, constipation, kidney stones and urinary tract infections. Nobody would want any of these ailments to strike in the best of times, so just imagine how nice it will be to minimize your risk of these occurring after gridcrash or in some other scenario (like travel or camping) when care may not be easy to find.

A final benefit of water for health has to do with respiratory infections. There is some evidence that staying hydrated protects you from viral respiratory infections and also helps people with asthma control their symptoms.

We have already talked about the importance of exercise and fitness in order to be adaptable to a future shift and to thrive after gridcrash. Exercise can also help prevent or control many of the chronic diseases (diabetes, high blood pressure, elevated cholesterol, heart disease, arthritis, cancer and depression, among others) that are the bane of modern life, even in the developing world. Again, even if you think all this talk of gridcrash is exaggerated, I hope I have convinced you of the utility and benefits of these lifestyle changes. Nowhere is this more important than with exercise: Modest exercise, like one hour of brisk walking each week, proved enough in most studies to have significant positive impact on your health. As noted above, though, I think you should be seeking a higher level of functional fitness than this.

Inactivity has been found to be just as dangerous as a moderate level of cigarette smoking. And it's almost never too late to reap the benefits of exercise. Even if you have emphysema, diabetes or coronary artery disease, for example, you can extend your life and improve your years' quality by improving your fitness.

Finally, as you go through all the efforts to get ready, don't forget to rest. In our rush-rush-rush Crackberry Facebook 24-hour news cycle text-messaging world many people don't get enough rest. We know that those who don't get enough sleep are at higher risk for cancer, chronic disease, obesity and injury. A recent study showed that those who sleep less than 7 hours per night have 3 times the risk of getting a cold after being given a dose of rhinovirus, one of the causes of the common cold, than those who sleep 8 hours a night. Even resting in bed while not sleeping did not confer the benefit of sleep.

The good news is that exercise alone helps improve both how much *and* how well you sleep when you go to bed. How cool is that: All of this stuff ties together. Drinking water may reduce your weight, exercise improves your sleep, and all of these changes will improve your health!

Conclusion:

Despite optimism in some quarters that we have seen the end of history, it is clear we live in turbulent times. The recent economic roller-coaster, climate change fears, potential energy insecurity and any number of other news items show that we can't simply rely upon naive optimism. It pays to make your life ready for gridcrash, but not just because of a post-crash world; you can derive benefits from your own efforts to make your body ready. If you don't want to do these things for cynical or selfish reasons alone, recognize that these activities can also reduce the impact your life exerts on others and on the Earth. For all of these reasons, now is the time to make your body ready: Get fit, get rid of your vices, and get yourself on a good diet with plenty of water. Then get a good night's rest!

Make Your Mind Ready

SELF-SUFFICIENCY IN ANY ARENA DEMANDS THAT YOU HAVE KNOWLEDGE AND SKILLS TO apply to activities needed for daily living. For many of these activities, the knowledge you need is easy to acquire, and for some areas, you already have much of the knowledge. You may have hobbies that give you skills that bear on sustainability. You may be a green-thumb, for instance, a master at raising flowers. This knowledge could be easily adapted to use in growing vegetables for helping to feed your family.

Other areas of knowledge needed for self-sufficiency are more esoteric and less commonly studied avocationally. Health care is certainly one of these areas. Few people read anatomy and physiology for fun. Instead, we rely on those further up the health care pyramid to use their interests and aptitudes to help us.

This chapter will guide you through some ways in which you can begin to acquire knowledge and skills in health care. As with most issues related to self-sufficiency, it is entirely up to you to decide how deep and broad you want these skills to be. For some, knowing simple first aid and hygiene measures will suffice. Others want more advanced skills, perhaps at the level of a nurse or EMT. A few will seek to gain credentials akin to an independent practitioner like a physician, an NP (nurse practitioner) or a PA (Physician Assistant) (PA). All of these are laudable goals.

Additionally, I will show you how you can use a community or neighborhood coalition, or "Village University." approach to train yourself and those close to you in obtaining these skills using experts that may already be among your circle of friends.

Finally, new media tools like the Internet, YouTube and iTunes make acquisition of skills in self-sufficiency cheap and easily accessible without having to attend classes or pay for materials or instruction. I will show you some of these to get you started "surfing the web" and will also talk about other ways of getting some training on the cheap.

Credentials vs. Competencies

FOR STARTERS, WE NEED TO EXAMINE THE GOALS YOU HAVE IN GETTING TRAINING AND KNOWLedge in health care. This is a key matter that is not an issue in most other areas of sustainable living.

Credentials basically allow you to add initials to your title: EMT, PA, RN, NP, MD, etc. They convey to others that you have engaged in the training and experiences needed to acquire competency in a field of knowledge, and that you have demonstrated competency in that field of knowledge to a degree that a licensing body (state or national) allows you to practice the skills appropriate to that credential.

You can develop competency equivalent to a lot of the credentials in health care without getting credentialed, but woe betide you if you attempt to use that competency but don't do it by the book with appropriate licensing. I am NOT suggesting that you try to practice without a license.

There are some people who argue, compellingly, that we have a right to self-treatment, and that the government monopoly on licensing creates a "cartel" that forces us to pay higher prices and forego other forms of treatment. Keep in mind that if you rely on the government or someone else to provide your health care, you get what they want you to have. You also get it only when they are willing and able to provide it.

Consider, for example, that you live in central Missouri and let's say that the New Madrid earthquake fault lets loose, as some are saying it will soon. Roads, power grids and waterways are all inoperable. Buildings in cities are damaged, some even collapsing. Your neighborhood has houses down, too, and trees litter roadways.

Under these circumstances, waiting for credentialed providers to come rapidly will be misguided. You will be on your own. The federal government may take days to arrive with help: Look at what happened after Hurricane Katrina in New Orleans. You may not have the credentials, but I hope you have the competencies should you find yourself facing one of these events.

In fact, Dr. Peter Safar, one of the inventors of CPR, said 20 years ago that *every household* should be able to provide six basic rescue and first aid skills *for itself* in the event of an earthquake. Can yours?

Basic Rescue and First Aid Skills

1. Airway control
2. Mouth-to-mouth rescue breathing
3. External bleeding control by compression
4. Recovery position
5. Shock position
6. Rescue pull

A look at the 2003 earthquake in Bam, Iran showed that 90% of initial care that was provided to survivors was given by family and neighbors. It took on average 1 hour and 45 minutes for credentialed rescuers to arrive at the side of the quake victims. Unfortunately, 90% of these friends and families did *nothing* for their loved ones, which led many to suffer and some to die, needlessly.

So, when I recommend that you obtain competencies, I don't expect that you get credentialed to practice them under normal circumstances in exchange for a fee. If you choose to do so, more power to you. I do hope that you at least obtain (and maintain) competencies to protect, maintain and restore health when the usual infrastructure, discussed in the introduction, is down.

Some writers (Aric McBay, Zachary Nowak, and Howard Kunstler, among others) think that things will soon be getting much worse. Rather than a discrete disaster, contained in time and scope, they foresee a gradual decline when we will be largely on our own in all areas needed to sustain life. Sending someone to find a professional with the needed credentials may be giving them a fool's errand under those circumstances; now is the time to make sure you have as many competencies as you can acquire in order to replace those with the credentials.

Acquiring Knowledge and Skills

TRADITIONAL SOURCES ARE GREAT PLACES TO START ON YOUR JOURNEY TO SELF-SUFFICIENT health care competency. Some cost real money—colleges and tech schools, for example. Others, like the Red Cross and some government agencies, only cost a little more than the time and energy you invest in the course. In these austere economic times for most families, I'd suggest you optimize your use of inexpensive resources, so we'll start there.

If you have not recently had first aid training, start by contacting your local Red Cross chapter. Most countries have offices, and larger countries will have them in several larger cites. Find out about taking a basic Red Cross First Aid course for about $50 or so. You can find out if you are motivated and interested enough to pursue further health care training; if you aren't, you will at least know more than when you started and can avoid having to worry that a Bam-like scenario might occur to your family. These courses are taught by lay people, and you could also further your own skills by becoming an instructor if interested.

Speaking of families: Take yours with you. Most older kids can handle the curriculum, and there are specific courses for youth as well. Bring your friends and neighbors, too. This would be a gentle introduction for them to the idea of starting down the sustainability trail with you.

The Red Cross also teaches CPR and a number of other useful courses like wilderness first responder and pet first aid, and they have a wealth of useful materials on their websites for free download that will help with disaster preparedness in general, in addition to first aid.

As noted above, other countries have the Red Cross or Red Crescent. Check out the website for the International Committee of the Red Cross/ Crescent to find your local or national office. There are also a number of useful publications on the ICRC site available for free download.

English-speaking countries of the former British Empire also are likely to have an active St John Ambulance Association that teaches similar courses. Look at their website for your country.

Another potential source of low-cost training in the US is the American Heart Association, which teaches basic CPR and some first aid courses that may be helpful to the neophyte, including some online versions. Many of these are geared to be taught in the workplace; maybe you and some coworkers can see if your boss will host a course. Having this training for employees may lower the insurance cost for the business and get you started for free.

In the United States, the federal government used to teach a medical self-help course as part of the civil defense efforts in the Cold War era. This course, like the Cold War that spawned it, has faded into the past, but the US government still has agencies that teach useful courses, often online and for free. (You can still download the manuals for the medical self-help course from the Federation of American Scientists website for interesting, although somewhat dated, reading.)

Now, the Federal Emergency Management Agency (FEMA), the Department of Homeland Security (HLS) via its website, and the Department of Health and Human Services (HHS) are the repositories of the tradition of the Medical Self-Help Course.

FEMA offers a number of courses for free on its website. In addition, if you are willing to invest the time and effort, the Citizens' Corps with its "Community Emergency Response Team" or CERT concept offers excellent training in disaster response, including disaster medical and stress response, as well as rescue and fire suppression. If you have a neighborhood, work or family-based group banding together for self-sufficiency, this would be an excellent starting point for a few dedicated individuals. Be aware, though, that the expectation is that you be available to the whole community in the event of a disaster.

Similarly, if you live in a small town or rural area, volunteering to be an EMT for the local volunteer fire or EMS agency may be an avenue to allow you to get some basic skills and supplies for only the cost of the time you devote to the training, plus the obligation of service you agree to when you join. You also will get to use your skills for real, and other advanced courses will open up to you. If you have more time and flexibility in your schedule and lifestyle, and money is a significant concern, CERT or volunteering are attractive options.

The next tier of training courses are offered to the public by private groups offering training in areas like "Wilderness EMT." "Wilderness First Responder." "tactical medicine" or "operational medicine." Google searches for any of these terms will turn up a plethora of potential vendors. Many are offered with law enforcement and military contracts in mind, but most will take unaffiliated students as well. Be aware that *caveat emptor* applies: You may not get what you pay for, so make sure you find someone reputable that has been teaching for a while and is not just taking advantage of the recent trend. Keep in mind, too, that some of these are directed toward the hard-core survivalist type, and while the information presented may still be useful and accurate, the delivery style may not appeal to you.

Another similar avenue, and one that may be more applicable to a crash scenario as we'll discuss later, is *maritime medicine*. Most of these courses last about 1 week. They are designed for those who truly live the title of this book as they cross big bodies of water without a physician or hospital nearby or easily reached. Talk about being self-reliant!

Both the land-based and maritime medicine courses cost more. You pay tuition, and may need to pay for supplies, above and beyond travel and lodging. Some are offered in nice resort locales, so you pay for that, too. As most courses run for several days, time away from home and work also factor into the burden. Again, if you have formed an intentional community to support neighborhood or family sustainability, this (like CERT) may be a place to send your key designated medical person.

Taking it to the next level, your local university, community college or technical college may offer EMT classes, nursing degrees and other advanced courses. In most cases, the expectation is that you are seeking the credential, not just competency in the subject. There will likely be less flexibility in terms of scheduling than with some of the courses listed above, and admissions requirements and cost become an issue as well. For instance, nursing schools will have prerequisites like chemistry courses that will add to the time and financial commitment of this route. Because of this, you may want to consider this route for a member of your family or group with clearly demonstrated commitment and aptitude for the health care subject area.

Other avenues to obtain training are out there. Brainstorm and let your fingers do the walking, via the internet. Look at your local, state and county medical societies, Rotary and other service organizations, and your local hospital websites to see if they are hosting courses of interest.

A hospital or other organization in your area doing continuing education, may sometimes need "victims" who agree to act out the roll of the sick and injured. Easy now: They don't require you to be sick or injured, but they may "moulage" you with makeup so you appear to have hideous injuries that disappear at the end of the day. When you volunteer, ask if you can audit the course in exchange for volunteering. Make it clear you are doing this for interest and edification only, and to make you a better victim, not as a back door to the credential. They may even be willing to let you have extra handouts or borrow course texts as well. Courses like Basic and Advanced Trauma Life Support fall into this realm.

Medical Auxiliary Model for Sustainable Health care

MEDICAL EDUCATION LEADING TO A DOCTORAL DEGREE IN MEDICINE (MD OR DO) IS A LONG road and is likely inaccessible to most people without causing significant upheaval in their current lives. In part this is due to the long preclinical or "basic science" phase of the first two years of medical school. Physician assistant school is shorter, only two years, but most PA programs require you to have a bachelor's degree, and others that you also have experience in a health care field, before entry into training. Nurse practitioners need a nursing degree prior to entering NP school.

Authorities in Great Britain have recognized that there is a lot of basic science knowledge in medical education's first two years that is never used by most physicians, according to the 2003 report "Tomorrow's Doctors". Public health and prevention, as well as listening and other communication skills are neglected. Still, there needs to be a foundation of some basic information like anatomy and physiology in order to maximize chances of accurate diagnosis and effective treatment.

Medical auxiliaries are trained for use in many parts of the world to work in places where physicians don't or won't work. (See *Barefoot Doctors and Medical Auxiliaries*.) They all share the common theme that they are non-physician clinicians trained over a shorter course than the 8-10 years required to train physicians, but they provide many of the same services as physicians.

TIP — **Barefoot Doctors and Medical Auxiliaries**

FOR MANY CENTURIES, NON-PHYSICIAN MEDICAL AUXILIARIES HAVE BEEN PROVIDING health care delivery in other countries, carrying out functions usually found under the scope of physician practice. In many cases, these auxiliaries have grown out of military practice, economic austerity or political upheaval. The current professions of nurse practitioner and physician assistant are the more modern, Western evolution of this concept.

Feldshers, perhaps the first recognizable auxiliaries, appeared in Europe in the 17th century. The concept probably originated in Germany, but flourished in the Russian military system under Peter the Great.

After training, the feldsher performed many physician functions, such as diagnosing and treating minor injuries and common illnesses. Many settled in rural areas of Russia and continued healthcare practice after ending service in the military; some even served in Alaska in the 1800s. The Soviet regime stopped training feldshers in the 1920s, but resumed it in 1937. Present day feldshers continue to serve in underserved areas of central Asia and some former Soviet Republics.

China trained more than 1.3 million *barefoot doctors* in the mid-1960s when physician training, along with other university education, stalled China during Mao's Cultural Revolution. These village-based auxiliaries received a 2-3 month training course; they learned by watching and listening to physicians. They also worked in hospital settings for additional supervision and training in Western medicine and the traditional Chinese arts of acupuncture and herb treatment. Initial training was interrupted by periods of military training and political indoctrination. Most worked in rural villages, applying public health measures to prevent common diseases.

The barefoot doctor was expected to get to know his co-workers and neighbors intimately. They were assigned to maintain immunization records, track the contraception methods used by women in the area, and arrange for consultation with a "real doctor" when necessary. Hygiene was another of the barefoot doctor's specialties. This personal approach helped improve the health of a nation considered backward because of poor public health and nutrition.

China still has about a million rural barefoot doctors who care for the country's hundreds of millions of rural farmers and peasants. Most of them have no formal medical education and little knowledge of Western medicine or how to use it. Mao's system was dismantled in the 1980s and '90s as China shifted the burden of paying for health care to individuals.

China's health authorities are using video-based distance education and other non-traditional education techniques to improve the skill level of these auxiliaries, and plan to have all barefoot doctors certified to a higher standard of training by 2010.

The barefoot doctor concept has most recently been applied in India, where women are trained as barefoot doctors to provide maternal and child health services to underserved women in their villages.

NOTE

One final model is the *clinical officer* concept, which has been used successfully in post-colonial Africa for many years. Doctors are only rarely trained in Africa, and many who study abroad stay behind in the US or Europe after their training has been completed. To help meet the shortfall of doctors, clinical officers are used. These medical practitioners have up to three years of training after high school. With this training, they are able to examine and diagnose patients, do minor surgeries, attend to pregnant mothers and the like. In fact, the only thing they don't really do is major surgery.

These experiences have shown that medical auxiliaries have a major role to play in health care delivery when physicians are not readily available, and that there are successful models outside the Western PA and NP credentials. These models can be applied to the village university concept to allow people to exercise their right to self-care.

In a gridcrash scenario, it makes sense to have continued access to health care even if access to physicians is not possible because of the situation. Having a level of skill approaching that of a medical auxiliary, built up slowly and as inexpensively as possible is one way of doing this.

As noted above, I am not suggesting you hang out your own shingle as a feldsher or clinical officer, as that would require that you take a recognized course to earn and be granted that credential, which may not even be recognized where you live.

Rather, I am suggesting that you develop the competencies that would allow you to function safely and effectively as the "barefoot doctor" for your "village" in the event that an earthquake, flood, war or similar widespread disaster disables the societal infrastructure.

Traditional and non-traditional routes all can be utilized to acquire the training needed to have the competency of a medical auxiliary, although you will have to work hard at innovative approaches in order to gain hands-on clinical experiences if you are not enrolled in a formal program. For these reasons, it may make more sense to ally yourself with someone working in health care already and appoint them your village doctor, as described below.

Non-traditional Approaches

NEW MEDIA, ESPECIALLY THE INTERNET, MAKE THE ACQUISITION OF KNOWLEDGE ONCE HELD closely by select professions much easier. Electronic courses via iTunes University for example, allow someone in the rural intermountain West to listen to lectures from Stanford, Cambridge and Yale, provided they have decent connectivity with the internet.

Books that are either out of print or that are not widely circulated, and may be prohibitively expensive for either reason, are now available for download via the web from a variety of sites. Many simply require that you register. You can download the classic books *Where There is No Doctor* and *Where There is No Dentist*, for example, among other useful volumes, at the Hesperian Foundation website just by registering your email.

A large number of the textbooks made available for free are relevant to a gridcrash scenario as many of them are collected for and directed at people who live in developing countries or serve in the military. Either of these situations closely approximates a post-crash scenario, so they are relevant.

There is a huge cache of health-related digital publications collected from various international and non-governmental organizations such as the World Health Organization and Doctors Without Borders. Finally, there is a wealth of information, primarily written for military health care providers, but useful nonetheless, for download from the Borden Institute.

If you are serious about becoming competent in gridcrash medicine so that you can care for yourself and those near and dear to you, it behooves you to become facile with accessing and using the medical resources available online.

Most of the resources you need will be available right from your home or work computer, but others like current medical, nursing and dental textbooks may require subscription services. In this case, you may find that a library at your local college or university has computer privileges you can use to access these materials, or you could also ask your local hospital if they have a library where you could access the material as well. Some larger public libraries may even subscribe to some of these services.

Many medical schools and large teaching hospitals have educational programs like community medical schools (where medical professionals give free lectures on medical subjects to the community at large) or Grand Rounds (weekly or monthly conferences given by subject-matter experts on wide-ranging medical and nursing topics). Surf the web to find out about what is available in your community.

Even agriculture colleges get in the act with some extension services having first aid, nutrition, health and disaster preparedness resources available at low or no cost.

Finally, you may be able to audit some health professions classes if you get permission from course directors. Find out if they need physical exam models, and they may let you listen in on the lectures teaching how these things are done; you may need to turn and cough, but they may even let you listen to lung and heart sounds with some basic coaching if you frame your request for information in the spirit of being a better model, as discussed above.

For hands-on experiences with procedures, you can make models for a number of procedures like inserting IVs, suturing wounds and the like; see *Cheap Models for Medical Procedure Training*. If you have a village university set up, some skills you need could be learned on other students as they learn on you. After all, countless nurses and doctors first practiced their skills on their classmates…

TIP ▸ Cheap Models for Medical Procedure Training

INSERTION OF INTRAVENOUS CATHETERS (IVs) IN ORDER TO GIVE A PERSON FLUIDS and medication is a basic nursing or medical technician-level procedure that many people involved in preparation activities focus on, with good reason. In the event of any number of illnesses or injuries that result in blood or fluid loss, the ability to resuscitate someone with IV fluid is potentially lifesaving. Medications may also need to be given intravenously, especially to unconscious patients or those with nausea and vomiting.

Another important activity, if you look at the lists of supplies and equipment recommended by preparedness-types, is suturing for repair of lacerations. We can anticipate that in an era when we are using manual tools or doing chores with our hands we will see more wounds, so this, too is a reasonable skill to acquire.

How can you learn how to do these things without having access to live patients? Models have been used for many years to provide this type of practice and training. When you couple old-school models with newer technology like YouTube and iTunes, you can add tremendously to the effectiveness of your Village University. There are lots of other models out there, and more are being developed all the time. If you have a particular skill you want to learn, look online to find potential models to help you master your art.

Gelatin IV Model

Most nurses, physicians and medical technicians recall the first time they started an IV on a living person. Many of us "got" to practice on our classmates, and have them practice on us, often with only a quick look at a video or after watching a live demo by the instructor. There may have also been a model provided. Unfortunately, these models were not very realistic: plastic arms that had track marks from so many previous sticks, and often fluid was seen leaking from their fake veins.

Advances in simulation for medical training have resulted in life-sized computer controlled manikins, but they are very expensive, making them unrealistic for small groups like a sustainability group.

A few years ago, Dr. Susan Stroud, one of my colleagues at the University of Utah Medical School, came up with an inexpensive, simple solution to the problem of training medical students to start IVs without having to bruise each other's arms and their own egos.

Dr. Stroud looked for models to help train her students, and finding no inexpensive model, made her own. Thus was the gelatin intravenous model (GIM) born. The GIM is easy to build out of readily available (and cheap) materials: a baking pan, real (not instant) gelatin and Penrose-type surgical drains tied off at the ends with "blood" inside. The GIM does not look like a junkie after a party: Its holes are self-sealing, preventing "bleeding" from the gelatin-encased "vein." Finally, the GIM responds more like human flesh than some of the more expensive, commercially made IV trainers. The gelatin gives a boggy, springy feel like real tissue under pressure, and the "veins" can roll like real ones.

At Yale University, a group of paramedic educators compared the GIM with traditional rubber arms for training neophytes. They found that the GIM is a viable alternative to training IV sticks using a human model and saves the trainees pain and pressure in learning this invasive procedure.

Now, many medical training programs use adjusted recipes to train resident physicians to put in specialized central IV lines or how to place an IV using ultrasound guidance. Other groups have replaced the flat baking pan with round tubular containers that they remove after the gelatin has set; this more accurately recreates the shapes of arms and legs.

Pigs Feet for Sewing?

Perhaps nothing is more de rigueur for the survivalist medic than to have a basic suture set. Knowing how to use it, though, is not always disclosed by proponents of having one of these kits available.

Most medical schools in the US nowadays seem to have at least one club- or curriculum-based lab that teaches interested students how to suture using pigs feet. As a medical educator, I too have made the trek to the butchers and endured the questioning looks as I picked up a few dozen fresh pigs feet in order to be able to teach suturing techniques to my charges.

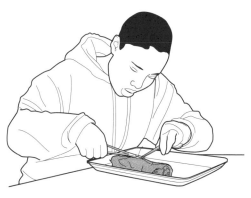

The benefit of this model is that pigs have thick skin, and you can create all manner of lacerations on their feet with a sharp scalpel. Then, you can sew to your heart's delight: Simple interrupted, simple running, mattress and corner stitches can all be practiced. You can also become a pro at basics like instrument ties, one method of securing the stitch with a sturdy knot.

One drawback of any model, such as the GIM or pig's feet, is that you can easily acquire the skills, but you will also need the cognitive background to allow you to apply them appropriately. One of my teachers in medical school used to say he could train a monkey how to do surgery, but learning when to do it took his human trainees many years. A good medical auxiliary will have both cognitive and procedural skills; don't overemphasize one set at the expense of the other.

The Village University: Learning the Skills You Need

PERHAPS THE LEAST CONVENTIONAL METHOD OF HELPING YOU ACQUIRE KNOWLEDGE IN GRID-crash medicine is the *village university* concept.

This book focuses on sustainability and helping you take care of yourself. Self-reliance only goes so far, though, as no one is an island. We can't count on being able to weather stormy times completely alone, so we need to look at ways to build relationships in our local communities that will help in our quest for sustainability.

In our post-industrial age, we have replaced community (and the compromise and relationships it requires) with technology. Like so many other areas of life, we don't often rely on our neighbors to provide assistance, nor they us. We seek a lifestyle that allows us to feed, clothe, shelter, entertain and care for ourselves "independently." In so doing we make ourselves dependent on technology, especially on cheap, readily available resources. We have seen that there is a cost to these cheap resources in that their use causes rippling impacts on the world's people and ecology.

In striving to lead a more sustainable life, you have to start with small, individual steps. In the end, however, community sustainability should be your goal: finding or forming a group of individuals that rely on each other more than on technology. The group will have to be interdependent within its walls, but ideally minimally dependent on external inputs.

What does it mean to be interdependent? In a gridcrash scenario, there are many activities needed daily for living that require special knowledge and skills. As much as we might idealize the image of the lone family or person out their making it alone, the breadth and depth of these needs are too much for any one person to acquire. Thus, we are best served by interdependence and a sensible division of specialized labor.

In fact, unlike the sustainability pyramid built on energy I described in the first chapter, I envision a different pyramid based on knowledge: At the base are simple skills and knowledge held by every mature member of the group, while further up, more specialized knowledge and skills are held by fewer people. There will be multiple pyramids for each of the areas of activity needed for sustainability: food procurement and storage, transportation, energy, shelter and health, for example.

Because of this, *you* may choose not to try to acquire advanced skills in health care for use after gridcrash, leaving that level of sophistication to others. Still, you must be able to do the basics in order to minimize your own illnesses and injury, as well as limiting the impact of those adversities on your group. You might be called on to help with basic care of others as well, just as you might consult someone else's superior knowledge and abilities in guiding activities like gardening or carpentry while doing the "grunt work" yourself.

The point is, within your group you should seek to identify someone most likely to be able to learn and apply knowledge and a set of skills to restore others to health. Others in the group may have some special training in medicine but won't emphasize it. If you are lucky, the lead person will already be trained and experienced: a physician, physician assistant or nurse practitioner, for example. Everyone has special skills and interests from work and hobbies; capitalize on these in choosing and allocating specialties within your group.

One way to spread skills is through the concept of a village university. This idea was popularized by three Scandinavian physicians working with victims of violence, especially landmine blasts, in the developing world. Basically, you bring in experts who then train select "village medics" within a community. After the initial training, the newly minted village medics train "helpers" who are deputized to help the medics. Often the helpers are from smaller collections of families living away from the main village.

You probably live in a neighborhood with a rich diversity of talents. If your neighbors are not interested in forming a sustainability group, maybe you can form one based on extended family and friends, coworkers, church members or others. If you live in a relatively large town or city, there is probably a peak oil or sustainability group already; you can go and maybe find like-minded members to help. Just do a web search with terms like *"peak oil"* or *sustainability*, plus the name of your town or city, and you are likely to find at least one such group.

Once you find or form your group, look at everyone's job and educational backgrounds. Then, think creatively: The insurance salesman may have been a medic in the military. The dentist or veterinarian will have a tremendous head start in learning more about human medicine. Most of those who have been to college may have taken classes in several fields before settling on a major or career direction; some may have changed careers after training in a health profession.

As you assemble a roster of knowledge and skills, keep in mind that some folks will have a job in one health field, but the training and experience acquired in pursuit and practice of their craft will stand them in good stead for training helpers in other areas. Trained health professionals can build upon their scope of practice and educational background to teach related areas.

Nurses, for example, do physical exams on patients and can teach basic assessment skills. Pharmacists know about drugs of course, but by necessity also know about microbiology and infectious diseases. Some know a lot about issues like treating patients after exposure to atomic, chemical or biological warfare. Other health care workers could teach skills relevant to their job;

a physical therapist could be very useful in teaching basic musculoskeletal anatomy, orthopedic and neurologic exams, and treatment of minor sprains, strains and fractures. These are just a few examples: Think creatively! You should encourage both building on old skills *and* using them to train other members of your community. Physicians are only really needed to train people in the most specialized topics.

If you don't have someone already trained as a health care professional in your group, you could sponsor someone to go through the training needed, like a medical auxiliary, starting with courses at the Red Cross and the like and gradually expanding to include CERT training or formal college-level courses. Many universities allow the option of auditing courses for adults at reduced cost; some are even free if you don't take the exams (and who would want to?).

The reality is that most folks don't have training or experience in taking care of sick and injured people. Most of the care required, though, is nursing care. A basic course in first-aid and basic safe nursing care, plus one in hygiene, will form the underpinning of further education, and will meet most needs. It forms the base of your health care sustainability pyramid.

Advanced courses in theory like physiology and pharmacology are nice, but may be a bit esoteric for a group trying to develop its own care team. If possible, your group should recruit a training nurse to help in this endeavor.

The only educational prerequisite for trainees is that they be interested, literate and numerate. Take advantage of free, public access materials like iTunesU and other resources found on the internet (see appendix) as your texts to minimize cost. You must make up a schedule that is realistic within your other life demands, with attainable goals. The curriculum should be focused on practical applications, covering essential materials using simple, straightforward terminology. A suggested curriculum is *Standards of Training, Certification and Watchkeeping for Seafarers,* required by the Coast Guard for the "Medical Person-in-Charge" (MPIC) providing health care on ocean-going vessels. An example of the items covered, which encompass more than simple bandage-and-splint first aid, is seen here.

Topics in the curriculum of the MPIC include:

- Suturing & Wound Care
- Intravenous Fluid Therapy
- Medication Administration & Injections
- Pain Management
- Infectious Diseases
- Behavioral Emergencies
- Eye, Ear, Nose & Throat

- Nasogastric Tubes & Urinary Catheterization
- Altered Mental States
- OB/GYN & Infant Care
- Complications of Drug & Alcohol Use
- Poisoning & Overdoses
- Legal Issues
- Communication & Documentation
- Anatomy
- Patient Assessment
- Respiratory Emergencies
- Cardiovascular Emergencies
- Defibrillation (AED) and CPR
- Bleeding & Shock
- Burns
- Environmental Emergencies
- Spinal Injuries
- Lifting & Moving Injured or Ill Patients

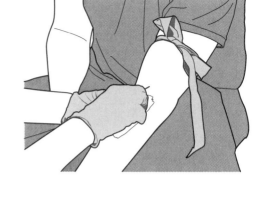

Clearly, this is a very comprehensive skill sets that (of necessity for seafarers) goes well beyond first aid. Whether you form a sustainability group or choose to go it more or less alone, you should strive to have someone trained at least to this level.

....

Conclusion:

Knowledge has been called power. Perhaps one reason for this is the realization that knowledge cannot be taken away. Time and biology can degrade knowledge slowly, but circumstances cannot take it from you once it has been acquired. Through recurrent training and practice you can reduce the effects of time on perishable knowledge. The physical and emotional fitness measures discussed in this book can keep your mind and body in optimal shape, helping to preserve your knowledge.

Gridcrash could potentially take many things away from you and your family, your community, region or nation. It may affect the entire world, like petrocollapse or climate change. In any case, the knowledge you develop prior to any crash will be useful before *and* after the crash. Rely on others to help you, as they will rely on you to make your family, neighborhood and community self-reliant. Devote time to learning what to do now, so you will have the skills when the time comes that you need them.

As we will talk about in the next section, what you know and how you act are at least as important as what you have.

Make Your Spirit Ready

EXPERTS HAVE TOLD US (AND EXPERIENCE HAS CONFIRMED) TIME AND TIME AGAIN THAT WHAT counts most in survival situations is not what you have, but how you think and behave. Although most of the work done in the psychological determinants of survival focuses on acute events like being lost in the wilderness, engaged in physical combat or held as a captive, we will focus on this body of work in light of gridcrash, as your spirit will bear heavily on your post-gridcrash life.

You are doing a lot to bolster your survival psychology just by reading this book. We know that people who have anticipated a bad event and thought about how it might affect them (and how they'd act in return) improve their odds of survival, even if they do nothing else. Surprise, and feeling overwhelmed because of it, can make you panic. Panic prevents clear thought and purposeful action, and it sets off a chain reaction that can lead you to do foolish things, or to do nothing. In a disaster, either course could be harmful.

What you are doing by reading this book and performing related tasks amounts to psychological *stress inoculation*. This is the idea of getting your emotional self ready for bad events. It is thus crucial for helping you to help yourself and others in bad times. This is true no matter how long those bad times may last: a minute, a day, or a year. Your forethought is a major element of this inoculation. Just like getting physically fit helps ready your body for physical rigors, so too does getting yourself emotionally fit make you ready for emotional stress.

The military and police as well as other first responders use stress inoculation. The goal of this technique is to expose people at risk for life-threatening danger to training that is so realistic that they are not overwhelmed by events when they occur in the real world. Even a "pre-briefing" before going into danger has been shown to help: Telling people about to be engulfed in a situation how it sounds, smells, looks and feels when they enter the fray has been shown to make them less prone to panic and allows them to be more effective.

In making preparations to safeguard your health and the health of those close to you, you are engaged in a form of stress inoculation. Later, we will talk about how to do medical threat assessments so you have an idea of what kind of emergencies you may face; others have written extensively about the wide variety of possible gridcrash scenarios and other disasters we may face. Taken together, this information can allow you to prepare for many eventualities. This planning, plus acquiring useful knowledge, skills and attitudes, will form the majority of the stress inoculation you need.

Stress inoculation may also help to reduce your vulnerability to the high rates of depression, substance abuse and PTSD found to occur after disasters like Hurricanes Andrew and Katrina. The World Health Organization defines a disaster as an event that overwhelms the *coping capacity* of a community. The techniques described here can help you bolster your coping capacity.

Additionally, there are other tools that have been used consistently by survivors that you should learn about now. Then, try to practice applying them in your mind in advance of trying times when you'll need them most. They are tools that could be useful in times other than just after gridcrash; they are applicable to any stressful and/or dangerous time you or your loved ones may encounter.

Traits of Survivors

SINCE THE SECOND WORLD WAR, A LOT HAS BEEN WRITTEN ABOUT SURVIVOR TRAITS THAT are less often found in those who don't survive similar conditions or circumstances. One classic arena in which these observations were made was in the POW camps of World War Two. Although the austere conditions in these camps were often due to a desire on the part of their captors to punish or torture prisoners, we can still learn a lot from the circumstances found there and the coping mechanisms used by some to help them survive.

Emotional stressors reported to affect these prisoners included shock at finding themselves in their new situation, depression in reaction to suddenly being in that situation, feelings of desertion or abandonment by their countrymen, uncertainty about day-to-day survival and how long they would be in their situation, and loss of self-respect. These psychological burdens compounded the physical deprivations forced upon them by hunger, exhaustion, cold, boredom and squalor.

According to the *Oxford Concise Dictionary of English Etymology*, disaster is derived from the Latin words for "unfavorable aspect of a star" and hails from a time when a person's star in the heavens protected them from bad events. As noted above, disasters can so overwhelm coping skills that it seems even the stars are against us. The principal psychological asset attributed to survivors is the nebulous "will" to survive or to live.

In the context of disasters like internment in a POW camp, the survivors, though bowed at times, did not wallow in the present. Instead, they refused to *feel* like prisoners, thinking of themselves as something else to support their will: as a father, a husband, an American or some other personal ideal. Through this technique, the survivors made conscious decisions to ignore or overlook their current straits and focus on the future. The past was their buttress of emotional support, not a burdensome reminder of better times. This view to the future was balanced and optimistic: A well-controlled "fantasy life" could be used to advantage. The exact nature of the diversion from the present was not so important and, when supported with hard work and courage, was not unrealistic or naive.

For the prisoners, this meant that they recited literature and poetry recalled from youth, taught and learned new foreign languages or had contests solving complex math problems, even at the risk of provoking the ire of their captors who tried to minimize contact among the prisoners.

Other experiences in these settings showed that physical illness and depression about circumstance became partners in a "negative feedback loop" where physical problems made emotional resistance weaken, allowing a worsening of physical illness and so on. Those who reacted realistically but optimistically and willfully against illness did better than those who seemed to give in.

Your Psychological Survival Kit

HOW DO PEOPLE REACT TO CRISES? THERE IS AN OLD SAYING THAT GOES ALONG THE LINE "There are some who make things happen, some who watch things happen and some who wonder what happened."

Studies into the behavior of people suddenly overcome by catastrophe show that 75% of these people are stunned and confused. At best, they resort to automatic behaviors and reflex action. Another 10% or so panic and give in to useless, inappropriate behaviors like screaming and crying or apathy. These two groups are the ones watching or wondering about events.

Only about 15% prove to be able to respond relatively calmly and are able to carry out useful activity. This small group makes things happen. Stress inoculation and a strong will to live may help keep you in, or move you into, this desirable demographic. . What other methods can be used to maximize your chances during catastrophe?

Journalist Laurence Gonzalez has written several popular books about the psychology of survival. His book *Deep Survival* describes how survival, regardless of the threat, can force upon us a journey. Those who survive seem to adopt a Zen-like acceptance of the journey and find a way to, if not enjoy it, at least not to fight it. He lists a number of patterns that survivors demonstrate in how they think and act. These patterns are not just directed towards outdoor recreators who may be lost and injured, and they can be condensed into a simple mnemonic device.

If you choose, you will learn (or may already know) that emergency care providers utilize mnemonics to help them recall critical actions in dire circumstances. A key mnemonic for these EMTs, nurses and physicians is ABC: Airway, Breathing and Circulation are priority functions that must be protected or restored.

For the survivor, the mnemonic ABCDEFG covers the keys:

A = Admission
B = Belief
C = Control
D = Discipline
E = Effort
F = Fun
G = Gift

These seven items, along with a strong will to live, will help maximize your chance of bringing yourself and those around you safely through any future shifts.

Gonzalez points out that survivors, ironically, go through the same five stages of grieving as patients given a terminal diagnosis, as described by Elizabeth Kübler-Ross. Denial, the first of these stages, can be deadly if it causes panic, inaction or the wrong action. Survivors move rapidly through denial with their *admission* of the difficulty of their circumstance to themselves. This does not mean they give in to hopelessness.

Psychologist John Leach has a name for this denial: *incredulity response.* Sometimes events like the building damage and collapse in the events of 9/11 are so overwhelming and out of the ordinary that some people simply can't or don't believe what they're seeing. They react with what is known as "normalcy bias" by trying to shoehorn the unusual events into the normal run of life. This often leads people to underestimate the danger they face up to the end, or at least until things have gotten so bad that they are in a real pinch. Some of us have seen how this denial occurs in those patients with a lump on the skin that grows and eventually disfigures them before they seek care.

Cancer patients and the doctors and others who care for them understand the power of naming. Learning that the nagging feeling you have is in fact due to cancer, although potentially devastating news, can in fact be liberating. Now, you have a focus for your emotions and your actions. What matters now is how you respond, not the event. The event has occurred and you alone determine how it will affect you.

Belief in themselves prevents survivors from being swallowed by despair. Not, as we saw with POWs, a pie-in-the-sky magical thinking, but capitalizing on self-knowledge of their abilities and their belief in the possible.

We are constantly regaled with stories of superhuman efforts that result in survival under staggering travails: people surviving on rainwater and a few fish for months at sea, or crawling deliriously for miles on injured limbs in freezing cold. All of these sagas share a dogged belief by those who live to tell them. that they will survive.

Many survivors describe how, after they have admitted to themselves the gravity of their position, they became either afraid or angry, or both. There must be *Control* of that anger and fear; indeed, once controlled, these emotions can be used productively as motivators. The adrenaline released in a "fright, flight or fight" situation will help you see and hear threats around you, and give you increased physical capacity, among other effects. Similarly, the anger or fear you feel, if directed appropriately, can allow you to perform better.

World War II prisoners described how they applied psychological first aid when they used "tough love" to keep their fellow detainees alive: They often used "systematic prodding" on those who seemed to be giving up. The anger thus induced in the subjects of the prodding frequently turned them around. (See *Psychological First Aid*.)

Psychological First Aid   TIP

PSYCHOLOGICAL FIRST AID (PFA, ALSO CALLED MENTAL HEALTH FIRST AID) IS A TOOL first developed back in the "Duck and Cover" days of the Cold War and Civil Defense. PFA might be needed anywhere traditional "physical" first aid is required.

Beginning in 1954, the American Psychiatric Association wanted the lay public to have the ability to help themselves, plus their loved ones and neighbors, to respond to the psychological consequences of disasters, including global thermonuclear war. The goal was to minimize the *disaster syndrome*, which afflicts so many after sudden devastation and prevents useful action. Another goal is to reduce feelings of help-lessness that might lead to PTSD or depression.

PFA is not designed to turn you into a counselor or a psychiatrist. It is a collection of tools to help you provide compassion and support to reduce the emotional impact of a stressful life event. This is some-thing we all do to a degree for ourselves and loved ones on almost a daily basis.

Most people who live through a disaster are affected emotionally by the event, but are not in need formal psychological help because of those effects. What people do need is protection from further harm, plus comfort, support and information. For some, protection means not having to relive the experience by recounting it, though others may find it supportive to talk about the events with other survivors. In any event, becoming physically "worked up" by talking about the event can cause further harm and should be avoided.

Next, comfort and support are provided. For most cases, this means reunification with loved ones, plus shelter, warmth, nutrition and medical support (if needed). Allowing "venting" of emotions may also help; some folks just want to know that someone is listening. The person giving PFA should appear confident, concerned and compassionate. Some survivors may find that channeling energy into productive activity is most helpful for their recovery from disaster emotionally, not to mention practically.

Finally, most survivors want information: about their loved ones and neighbors affected by the disaster, about the future and the like. This should be reliable information only, not rumor or speculation.

The last tenet of PFA that must be remembered is that, just like in first aid given for illness or injury, some folks will need professional help. Those with dysfunction (who can't eat, sleep, talk or care for them-selves or loved ones, for example) are those most at risk for PTSD and will benefit from referral to professional help as soon as it is available.

See "Psychological First Aid for First Responders" available at mentalhealth.samhsa.gov/disasterrelief/pubs/manemotion.asp for more information on disaster psychology services. There is a free downloadable course manual covering mental health first aid available to interested readers for more PFA information; see the resources at the end of the book.

Discipline-led action must become the product of your use of Admission, Belief and Control: organized, planned and deliberate efforts to allow you to over-come the survival situation. Hikers who are lost but uninjured often succumb to exhaustion and cold from denial and panic-driven efforts to find a way out. Survivors recognize the situation, know that they are likely to be rescued, control their emotions and set about to build shelter and a fire to protect themselves.

Sometimes discipline takes the form of *active passiveness*. Active passiveness is deliberate inaction: "Don't just do something, stand there." This passiveness may last just for a blink—only pausing to check where the fire is, then going in the direction needed to get away. Those who don't take this pause may paradoxically head toward the threat.

Other times, active passiveness is a state of mind where you force yourself simply to be present without responding emotionally to the circumstance. This is part of the idea of a Zen-like state, accepting fate with equanimity.

Once you have your plan, you must apply *Effort* to make the plan into reality. This is a key component of making your belief in yourself real, rather than mythical. Cancer survivors describe learning to value the pain they endured in their treatments, embracing it as the effort required to get better. Darrell Stingley, a New England Patriot's receiver paralyzed in a game reportedly spoke to this when he said "Pain is your friend" because it signaled a welcome return of sensation as he went through his rehab.

Gridcrash may not sound like a good time to any sane person, yet survivors have shown that having *Fun* is essential to keeping going. Small victories, pleasant surroundings, and finding humor in the absurdity of the situation, among other treats, provide the source of that fun for countless survivors.

Finally, as another part of the Zen-like journey, comes the *Gift*. Survivors recognize that they will learn much about themselves from their triumph over each obstacle. That is treated as a gift in and of itself. Others focus, despite their trial, on the well-being of others: Helping those with you, and thinking of loved ones apart from you, can take the focus away from your burden and help boost morale.

Leach, in his book *Survival Psychology*, describes how caregivers in disasters have higher rates of survival, as they did in the concentration camps and Gulags of Europe in the recent past; perhaps this is in part due to their focus on making things a little better for others.

Conclusion:

Austere conditions due to economic collapse, natural disaster, or any number of other problems could put us into circumstances similar to those described above.

Surviving and flourishing in any situation requires not only tools, supplies, physical ability and cognitive knowledge, but also (and perhaps most crucially) attitude. Your preparations in other "meatier" or more practical realms like fitness and medical training are essential; these will help your psychological preparation as well. Carrying a strong will to live, plus keeping a psychological survival kit containing the *ABCs* of a strong survival mindset, will take you a long way under any shift in circumstances the future may bring your way. ●

CHAPTER 3

Planning

Planning

HOPEFULLY, THE FACT THAT YOU HAVE MADE IT THIS FAR INTO THE BOOK MEANS YOU ARE convinced that what you know and how you behave are much more important than any thing you have stored, made or purchased over the years. Having said that, this chapter will cover some of the planning that you need to do in terms of things you need to acquire, make or otherwise have on hand in the event of a crash.

Preparation for gridcrash makes sense because it is applicable to ordinary times, or at least to extraordinary events during ordinary times.

This chapter includes discussion of several important topics:

- first aid kits
- medications
- sickrooms
- special needs populations
- neighborhood/community preparedness
- influence of climate, geography, and other factors

First Aid Kits

I FREQUENTLY EMPHASIZE THAT THE PREPARATIONS DESCRIBED IN THIS BOOK ARE USEFUL FOR real, everyday life. I am hoping that, as we talked about in terms of getting your mind ready for the crash, you see the logic of at least having simple first aid supplies on hand. Accidents happen everyday to ordinary people.

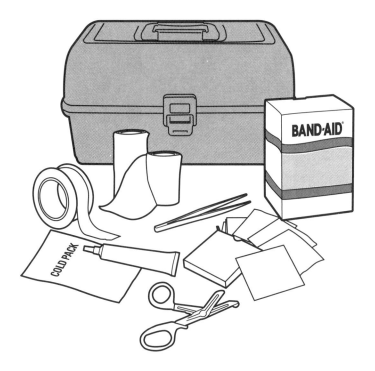

Just like having a Stradivarius when you're not a concert violinist doesn't make much sense (except perhaps for rich collectors), you don't need a top-of-the-line medical kit, but rather just some simple supplies. For starters, you should have simple bandages and other items that will allow you to do "bandage and splint" type first aid.

You should have these items available in places where you're likely to need them: at home, in your car, in recreational vehicles, and at work (if not provided by your employer). Obviously the kits for portable use are of necessity going to be smaller and perhaps less complete than the one at home.

One thing that every first aid kit (FAK) must have, even if you have nothing else, is personal protective equipment (PPE). We live in a day when blood-borne pathogens like hepatitis and HIV are commonplace in the community, and many people don't know or won't tell you if they have these infections. If you choose to be a Good Samaritan and render assistance, you should be able to at least protect yourself and thereby your family. This makes having simple items like nitrile or latex gloves, plus possibly spray shields and masks to cover your eyes and mouth, respectively, essential. I work in health care and have seen all manner of what strike many folks as gory things. Still, getting somebody's blood or other body fluid on me is pretty unappealing, even if it is uninfected, to say nothing of a potential infection source. We will cover PPE in more detail in the next chapter.

Beyond that consideration, first aid kits are a lot like diets; I will leave it largely to your discretion to determine what you need. I provide some suggestions which you can modify according to your situation, your level of training and comfort in providing first aid, and your concern about the need to be able to render more advanced medical care.

There are huge numbers of vendors willing to sell you first aid kits. Many of these kits are excellent while others may be less so. Many contain exotic items that you may never use, and others may lack items that you need more routinely.

In addition, keep in mind that in a disaster situation, the *Field of Dreams* phenomenon applies: "If you build it, they will come," meaning if you demonstrate that you are prepared by having supplies and knowledge, don't be surprised if word gets out. In the aftermath of Hurricane Katrina, many families who offered shelter and other services to friends and strangers were overwhelmed; some have written blogs that strongly recommend that you have extra supplies available.

In addition to off-the-shelf first aid kits, you can find custom FAK builders online (see the appendix for a list of potential vendors). To me, it makes sense to build your own first aid kit. In doing so, you'll have much more control over what you have on hand, and you can choose supplies that are appropriate to your situation. In many cases, this is also a less expensive route. You can also have control over the type of container used for the kit. Some people simply use large ziplock-type bags in which they hold the FAKs in their car, whereas others go for a full-on dedicated sturdy box, like a fishing tackle box.

In the tables in this chapter, I have adopted recommendations of organizations like the American Red Cross and the American College of Emergency Physicians to compose a suggested list of items for a home FAK as a starting point for you. Other books like *Preparedness Now* (from the Process Media Self-Reliance Series) contain suggested lists of basic first aid supplies, and I think they are very reasonable. The appendix for this chapter will have more FAK suggestions.

Keep in mind that as you grow in experience and training, and make the decision to be in a position to provide more advanced care like suturing wounds, you may need other items that are available through medical supply stores and even eBay. (See *First Aid Kit Items on eBay*.)

INTERNET AUCTION SITES LIKE EBAY HAVE PROLIFERATED OVER THE LAST FEW YEARS. To the person interested in sustainability, or the group forming a sustainability coalition, these sites offer the opportunity to obtain a number of supplies at low cost.

On a single day, with just a few minutes of surfing on eBay, I was able to find the following items to stock a FAK and/or sickroom:

- Resuscitation bags and masks
- CPR barrier mask
- Surgical face masks with plastic shield (protects eyes)
- Nitrile and latex gloves
- N95 masks
- Tivek suits
- EMT bandage ("trauma") shears
- Kerlix and Kling Gauze Roller Bandages
- Cobam self-adherent dressing
- Antibiotic ointment packets
- Tourniquets and Hemostatic agents
- Malleable (SAM) splints and Ace-type elastic bandages

NOTE

You can also find other items likely to be useful for a large group intending to train and equip their own medical auxiliary. These items are often available at lower than usual cost via eBay. Often you can find supplies in large lots.

Be aware because many items are sold as-is; make sure that their packaging is still intact, especially in the case of sterile supplies. Some items are also somewhat perishable and may have short expiration dates. Some I've seen sold have even been listed despite being out of date. Caveat emptor!

In addition, remember that many household items can be adapted for use in first aid, and a number of medical items have multiple uses for innovative, imaginative providers. (See *Household Items for First Aid*.)

This is especially so in cases of severe austerity. I will talk more about what to have in a more advanced kit for a true "when there is no doctor" scenario in Chapter 5 of this book.

First aid kits are listed among the "Ten Essentials" for a simple reason: When you need one, you need one! Always have at least a basic one with you at work or in your car, and a more complete kit at home.

Household Items for First Aid TIP

YOU SHOULD TRY TO HAVE A GOOD FIRST AID KIT NEARLY ANYWHERE YOU GO, BUT when you don't, you may need to improvise some things for first aid from household items. Obviously this is less than ideal. Here are some suggested items found in many houses that could help in a pinch when put to a different use:

Plastic bags: Place over your hands for improvised gloves; fill with ice for an ice pack; fill with water, then puncture with a safety pin to make a pressure-irrigation system for cleaning a wound or rinsing out an eye.
Saran Wrap: Cover a bad burn to help lessen pain and reduce infection risk (a University of Iowa study showed this was safe and effective).
Tampons: Place a new tampon in deep wounds to form a pressure dressing (the tampon expands to compress, or tamponade, the bleeding site).
Any clean cloth (bed linens, T-shirts, etc.): Use in place of gauze as a dressing.
Duct tape: Useful for securing dressings and bandages.
Belts: Use to make a sling or secure a pressure dressing (be careful it's not too tight).
Newspapers or magazines: Rolled to make a tubular splint for a broken arm or leg.

There are undoubtedly many other household items that, in extremis, could double as first aid supplies with a little bit of imagination, but I would rather have a good FAK on hand so that I don't have to tear up my T-shirt or get my belt all bloody.

Medication Issues

WE KNOW THAT MOST OF THE MEDICATIONS PRESCRIBED IN THE US ARE PRODUCED OVERSEAS, primarily in Asia. There is a long supply chain to follow before a prescription written by a health care provider can reach the patient who takes the medicine, even if the pharmacy is just across town.

If you take any medications routinely for any kind of chronic illness, you should talk to your doctor (or other health care provider who prescribes them for you) now about the possibility of obtaining at least one month's worth of extra medication. If there is an interruption in that medication supply chain, for instance a problem importing medications from India or China, or other infrastructure disruption on a more local level, you may have enough of a medication on hand to make it through until the supply resumes, or to allow you to make other arrangements like changing medicines if needed.

Physicians would be willing to do this in most cases, perhaps excluding chronic narcotic pain medications or other mood altering substances. Your insurance company may not allow you to routinely purchase medication in advance using their benefits, so you may need to clear it with them first or pay out of pocket.

In austere circumstances, there are other potential sources for prescription medications, such as taking veterinary medications intended for animals, although this is generally not recommended. Read more about this in the final chapter.

Most medications last much longer than the expiration date listed on the packaging, provided that they are stored in good conditions (dry conditions, about room temperature and in the dark). Because of this, most of the extra medications that you need will last years and you can simply rotate the stock as needed. (See *Medication Shelf Life*.)

In addition to prescription medications, you should have on hand a supply of over-the-counter medicines for use on a routine basis in your home for minor illnesses and injuries.* This also needs to be age-specific, so that if you have children, you have liquid or chewable medications that are appropriate for the children in your life. Make sure these are medications that you tolerate, and ideally that work well for you, as you should know from experience by having taken them before. One suggested list is:

■ Painkiller/antipyretic (fever-lowering) medication
(best to have some of each)
- Acetaminophen (brand name is Feveral or Tylenol)
- Ibuprofen (Advil, Motrin, etc.)
- Naproxen (Aleve)
- Aspirin (not for routine use in kids due to Reye's Syndrome)

■ Gastrointestinal Agents
- Antacid medications (Tums, Rolaids or other chewable)
- Zantac, Prevacid or similar acid-blocker
- Immodium or similar antimotility diarrhea medicine
- Bismuth Subsalicylate (Pepto-Bismol)
- Rehydration solution like Pedialyte
(See *Fluid Administration without an IV* in Chapter 5;
- Could be homemade using Salt, Sugar, and Baking Soda)

■ Antimicrobial/wound-care agents
- Povidone iodine wipes (very effective and painless, but messy)
- Benzalkonium chloride (Bactine is one brand; helps limit pain)
- Isopropyl alcohol pads
- Antibiotic ointment (like Bacitracin, Neosporin, Polysporin)

■ Burn care
- Aloe Vera gel (used for burns and other various skin problems)
- Burn gel

■ Antihistamines (for allergic reactions, mild to severe)
- Diphenhydramine (brand name Benadryl)

■ EpiPen auto-injector (for those with life-threatening allergies)

■ Rash/topical anti-itch treatments
- 1% hydrocortisone cream
- Antihistamine cream (like Benadryl)
- Calamine or oatmeal-based lotion

■ Treatments for poisonings
- Activated charcoal (use as directed by poison control center)

*In the event of longer-term crash, or if you are seeking more natural health care methods, you may choose to learn about alternatives to pharmaceutical medications. See Chapter 5 for information on herbal medicine and food as medicine.

Medication Shelf Life

SURVEYS INDICATE THAT ALMOST HALF OF AMERICAN ADULTS HAVE USED A MEDICATION that has passed its expiration date, despite FDA recommendations to discard all medications, prescription as well as OTC, that hit their expiration date. Under routine daily life conditions, relying on an expired medication to help if you have a serious illness, rather than getting a fresh refill, is foolish.

What about after gridcrash? Nobody really knows the actual safe and effective shelf life for most medications. Most manufacturers generally use a two- to five-year window for their expiration dates, but not always due to either safety or effectiveness concerns. The FDA requires that the product will contain at least 90% of its original potency until the drug expires. The expectation is that the product is stored according to packaging directions with the original packaging unopened and intact.

Medications that are still in their original package from the maker when sold retain the manufacturer's expiration date. On the other hand, if a pharmacist repackages the drug into new containers, the prescription gets a new date: a use-by date or beyond-use date (BUD). In most cases, this will be one year from the time the prescription was issued, based on the US Pharmacopeia standards, or as determined by state regulation.

Doctors and drug companies generally are mum on this issue, primarily due to liability. The AMA has reported that most expiration dates are probably too short and recommended wider study of the issue to save on pharmaceutical costs.

Little data on medication shelf-life has been published, though most is promising. The biggest study is the FDA's Shelf Life Extension Program (SLEP), begun in 1985 to try to save on the cost of medications used by the government. The FDA tested drugs stockpiled by the military services as well as the VA, Coast Guard, and the Department of Health and Human Services. Potency and quality were studied on drugs that had been sitting around in warehouses. The FDA stresses that the SLEP was only intended for government-stockpiled medicines, but the lessons learned are useful for gridcrash aficionados.

There is dramatic variation in shelf life between manufactured lots of the same drug. That is just one reason why the SLEP states their results cannot be applied to retail drugs. Most people, for example, store medications in bathroom medicine cabinets, where high heat and high humidity conspire to create the worst conditions for stability and potency. Medicine stored in a place where heat and humidity are lower and steadier, like a basement, probably will retain potency longer.

Based in part on the report of the SLEP, plus a smattering of other studies, the Medical Letter, widely read by physicians and pharmacists, stated in 2002 that drugs stored in ideal conditions would be useful for more than 5 years after their expiration date!

While it is certainly better to err on the side of safety when it comes to drugs, keep in mind that under a long gridcrash scenario, you may be forced to choose to keep your medicines on hand for a rainy day, or face the alternative of throwing potentially lifesaving drugs away…

If you choose to purchase drugs for stockpiling, I recommend that you try to rotate stock so that they don't go out of date. Look for coupons to lower the cost of OTC medicines, and see if generic formulations are an option for your prescription medications.

Should you decide on trying to stock up on drugs and "unofficially" extend shelf lives, keep in mind the caveats of the SLEP—original packaging (ask your pharmacist to sell prescription medications in the blister packs or "stock bottles" from the manufacturer, if possible) and optimal storage conditions (cool*, dark and dry). Make sure to label your stocks appropriately, and whatever you do, make sure that children and pets CANNOT get at them! Finally, keep in mind that some drugs like nitroglycerine have short expiration dates due to loss of efficacy.

NOTE

Some drugs, especially liquids, may need refrigeration; see packaging for information on best conditions.

Sickrooms: A Relic of the Past You Should Consider

UNTIL JUST RECENTLY, MOST HOMES IN THE US AND MANY OTHER COUNTRIES HAD A SICK-room: a place where someone with a potentially communicable disease was lodged while ill. That was when the "old country doc" still did house calls and hospitals were usually reserved for those with no home and no family. Family members, usually women, acted as caregivers to the person in the sickroom and cared for them using skills and knowledge that the average responsible housewife was expected to have acquired by reading and talking to doctors.

The goal of isolation in the sick room, of course, was primarily to minimize contact between the sick person and those susceptible to contagion. With the advent of vaccines, disease eradication and antibiotics, sickrooms have become historical footnotes. In an age of gridcrash, they will become useful tools handed down from our forebears.

Why would you want a sickroom? I don't advocate having one room left vacant and otherwise unused for anticipated use as a sickroom. I do suggest you choose a room now where you *could* safely isolate an ill or potentially infectious family member. Why this distinction?

Well, let's say there is a severe influenza pandemic, and you have to keep working for economic, professional or ethical reasons. Because you may be exposed to folks who have the flu, you may not want to take the risk of exposing family members to the illness, which can be transmitted by people before they have flu symptoms. In this case, having a room at home where you can isolate yourself, but still be with your family, offers them some protection and simply makes sense.

Ideally, your sickroom would have its own entrance directly from outside, as well as its own bathroom. Good outside ventilation and natural sunlight are also important, as we will discuss in the next chapter. The goal is to allow those who work outside the home to have a place to come "home" to while allowing them to minimize contact with family members who have to stay at home.

What, stay home, you say?!? Keep in mind that many of the *social distancing measures* planned by the CDC to slow the spread of a flu pandemic include closing schools, malls and other places where large groups of people could congregate and exchange germs, as we saw in Mexico in Spring 2009 during the early days of swine flu.

In these circumstances, daycares will also be likely to close. We may get to a point where only "essential" services are working; if you happen to work in one of these services, you need a sickroom.

Another reason to have plans for a sickroom is that a time may come when we have to care for sick loved ones at home ourselves with minimal outside help. Most modern pandemic flu models predict that there will not be enough doctors, nurses, hospital beds and ventilators to treat all of those likely to be afflicted with influenza, even for a mild to moderately severe outbreak (like we saw in 1957 and again in 1968). There may be other previously unknown infections, as SARS recently showed us, which could cause similar problems. Many states are already anticipating using widespread homecare during a pandemic.

PANDEMIC SWINE FLU/NOVEL H1NI
United States Cases from the CDC

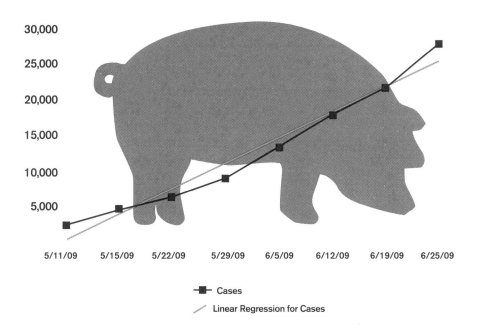

Finally, you may need to do *reverse isolation* where you keep a loved one with a weakened immune system (say due to chemotherapy for cancer) shielded from infection, perhaps from children, who sometimes seem to willingly share nothing *but* germs. Having a plan in place for a sickroom will be essential to allow this type of isolation.

We all remember the "plastic sheets and duct tape" days of the terrorism scares, but in the event of major concerns about infection in a family member or other cohabitant, it makes sense to be able to isolate this room from the rest of the house. (See the Department of Homeland Security website on "staying put" in the event of a pandemic for instructions on how to do this type of isolation. You will need to modify this so you can get some outside ventilation.)

This room should also be easy to clean. If the floor is carpeted, you may want to put down plastic sheets to allow you to disinfect the floor with bleach wipes. For the same reason, keep dirty clothes and soiled linens in the room until you can wash them in hot, soapy water, with bleach if possible. Hanging the wash outside in the sun for 8 hours will also help disinfect fabrics.

Minimize *fomites*, which are objects like books, dishes, etc. that can harbor infectious agents. You may want to have a supply of paper plates and other disposable dishes, too, to minimize having to wash dishes from the sickroom even though this may not exactly be ecologically sound. Furniture surfaces should also be suitable for wiping down with bleach.

The person in the sickroom will have a relatively monastic existence, taking meals and spending most time at home in the sickroom. No roaming around the house. Contact with other family members would be safest if one or both parties uses appropriate PPE. (see Chapter 4.)

You also should think about the morale of the person in the sickroom, whether actually sick or just at risk. Personal comfort items like snacks, books and magazines, (cheap and disposable, not first editions...), music, games and even a television, will make the rough times a bit more bearable.

Most of what you need to supply your room will be found easily in hardware or grocery stores.

A suggested list of items to have on hand for operation of a sickroom includes:

- N95 Respirators (N100 OK, too)
- Goggles or other eye shields
- Isolation gowns (full length, with full sleeves)
- Disposable "exam" gloves (nitrile to avoid latex allergies)
- Bleach: liquid (plain, unscented) and wipes; plan on having extra
- Spray bottles for bleach and/or other disinfectant solution (like Lysol)
- Trash cans, both inside and outside the room
- Antibacterial soap
- Waterless alcohol-based hand sanitizer gel
- Hand lotion (your hands will get dry from all the washing)
- Waterproof bed spread (preferably will cover the whole bed)
- Waterproof pillowcases
- Surgical masks (for patient wear; offer caregiver additional protection)
- Plastic sheeting (best is sheeting that is 2-4 mils thick for durability)
- Vent fan for negative air-flow (air comes *in* to room, not *out* to house)
- Dishware (consider disposables, or bleaching in room to sterilize)
- Water supply for the patient (tap in room, pitcher or bottled)
- White towels and linens (can be cleaned with bleach)
- Disposable bed pads (like Chux or similar blue pad, for bodily wastes)
- Big bucket or bin with lid (for holding soiled linens)
- UV Light Air Purifier (not filter)
- Bedpans and (for males) urinals
- Thermometer

- Comfort foods (candy, snack foods, etc.)
- Morale items (magazines, books, video games, etc.)
- Microwave oven
- Refrigerator (dorm or mini-bar size)
- Television and/or radio

We may again see the classic picture akin to those portrayed by Norman Rockwell of the caregiver checking the temperature of an ill child lying in bed at home. If you prepare now, your outcome should be just as rosy as that little boy's cheeks.

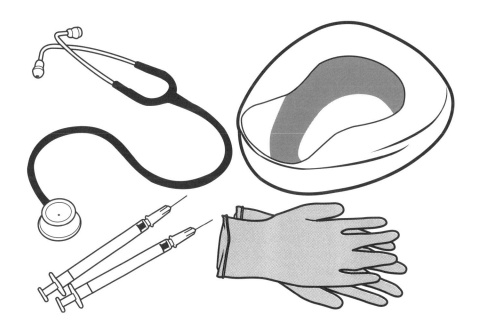

Special Needs Populations

IN 2004, THE CDC DEFINED SPECIAL NEEDS POPULATIONS AS THOSE "WITH DISABILITIES, people with serious mental illness, minority groups, the non-English speaking, children, the homeless, and the elderly." I also include in this group, for the purposes of disaster planning, those with other serious chronic health problems like diabetes, asthma, or high blood pressure, among others. Obviously this group could be huge, and we are all future or at least potential members of this group for one reason or another.

The major issue for special needs populations is that they usually have medical needs that are different from those of the general population. In terms of your planning and prevention activities before a gridcrash scenario occurs, much of the focus belongs on these special needs within your family. After gridcrash, people who have special health care needs may be largely on their own, along with the rest of us. If there is someone in your family who would have trouble planning or acting for themselves, work now to help them. If you know

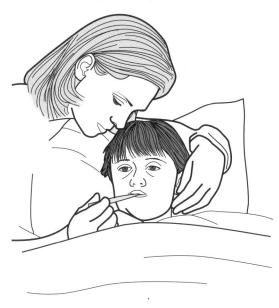

someone in the same situation, ask how you could help them through a disaster.

As the first step, we will focus on planning for a short-term, geographically limited disaster like a blizzard or hurricane. After that, we will look at ways to mitigate the effects of a "long emergency" type of situation on these folks.

Perhaps the first issue for those planning for someone with special needs to consider right now is evacuation: If a hurricane or other major weather event that would threaten your house were headed your way, you must know in advance when to leave, where you will go and how you will get there.

Most advocates recommend that anyone with mobility issues or other special needs plan to evacuate early, with the first notice, rather than waiting for a mandatory evacuation. This takes care of *when*.

Laws have required that local governments develop mass evacuation and departure plans for special needs groups. Despite this, a group studying this issue for the National Research Board reported in 2008 that most local plans did not meet the needs of the special needs population. You need to be sure to have a way of getting where you need to go; redundancy is important if you rely on others.

Once you are aware of how you are going to travel, be aware that many shelters set up after hurricanes or similar disasters are not designed for evacuees with special medical concerns. You must plan to bring any special equipment you need, like oxygen, wheelchairs, etc. with you.

Find out from the local or national voluntary organization specific to your special need or status if there is a registry for your area of people who need assistance in the event of a disaster. Your local, county or state health and human services agencies may also have similar registries. These groups should also be able to help you learn about shelters that are compatible with your particular special need.

If there is no registry specific to your needs, find out from these organizations how to go about forming one. The purpose of the registry is to collect and convey answers to the when, where and how questions above. Keep in mind that privacy will need protection; make sure that not just anyone can get access to the registry.

The smallest form of registry is a network for personal support: a group of several people you know in areas like home and work (places you spend a lot of time) who are willing to help you if disaster strikes.

Another consideration is the acquisition and storage of medications and other supplies required by special needs populations. Many of these will be chronic medications used on a routine basis for the elderly or those with chronic illnesses. Others include dosing forms needed by children or possibly special dosing forms needed by those unable to swallow, for instance, and therefore fed via tubes. The considerations discussed above in the section on medications are especially relevant for special needs populations.

You may also have durable medical equipment like corrective lenses, oxygen, CPAP machine, wheelchairs and the like. Make plans for manual back-up or other accommodations in case the lights go out.

Next, find out what might prevent you from accomplishing your activities of daily living on a near-normal basis after any disaster. Hospitals call this a "hazard vulnerability analysis." Non-governmental organizations like CARE and companies (including the military and police SWAT teams) who send folks overseas or into other austere environments talk about Medical Threat Assessments, which we will cover in more detail below.

Whatever you call it, do an assessment of your needs and the resources you rely on during normal times to meet them, then try to identify or brainstorm things in your area that might threaten them. Focus on things needed to sustain a minimally acceptable level of functioning of your daily activities, plus mobility issues.

Of course, all of the foregoing (with the possible exception of your personal network) could be compromised in a big disaster like Hurricane Katrina. This brings home the importance of having preparations in place and a network to help. You may have family who rely on you to be their network. In the event of a major infrastructure disruption, you and your network will experience the YOYO phenomenon: You're on your own!

Caring for folks with special needs will obviously be very difficult in the event of severe infrastructure collapse, but this does not mean you should throw your hands in up hopelessness and entirely forego planning and preparing. On the contrary: Get to work now!

Try to maximize body and spirit prep in these folks, too, not just in those with routine needs; obviously you will need some modification of these preps for some. Make especially sure that relevant immunizations are current in this group. Get to know disease management techniques for the disease(s) that affect you or them in case medicines and care providers are in short supply. These last two topics are coming up in the next chapter.

Disasters create special needs populations in the areas they strike. If gridcrash occurs, we will all have special needs. If you already know someone with special medical needs, or have them yourself, you need to make sure that the imposition of special needs due to circumstance does not overwhelm your ability to meet your routine needs. Planning and creative, realistic thinking now will help lower the chance of you becoming overwhelmed.

Planning for Your Pets

I INCLUDE PETS IN THIS CHAPTER BECAUSE MANY OF US CONSIDER PETS TO BE PART OF THE family. I will not have much to say about livestock, although if you live in a rural area, or plan on raising livestock as part of your sustainability efforts, you should consider training veterinary auxiliaries, analogous to the training of medical auxiliaries described in the last chapter. At minimum, a pet first aid course at your local American Red Cross chapter should be considered.

Remember that pets may not behave normally during or after a disaster; a lot of us have seen the nervous pacing of our dogs during the 4th of July neighborhood amateur fireworks contests. Pets that normally love their human or animal companions may fight, bite or otherwise act in unusual ways.

Next, consider that pets may flee during disaster. The changed landscape after some disasters may obscure the usual clues they rely on to find their way home. Make sure that animal control agencies can identify your pet so your family can be reunited. Find out if there is a shelter for pets where they can go in the event of an evacuation if you yourself are likely to end up in a shelter for people, as most state health laws do not allow human shelters to accept pets.

Keep your pet up to date on shots, just like you do yourself, because infectious diseases are rampant after disasters, and animal shelters won't take pets who haven't had their shots!

Make sure that your plans for sustainability include your pets, too: Have a kit for their basic needs, ideally one that is portable and ready to go in case you have to "bug out."

If you have to leave your pets behind, make sure that they are not too hot or cold and that they have access to food and fresh water. You could leave a faucet dripping into a dish, or use automated food and water dispensers. Your pets should also have places that they can go safely to eliminate wastes. An unfinished basement, a fenced backyard or porch or your garage may work best for these purposes.

Finally, remember that like we discussed above, a lot of the medicines we use are also made for animals. Keep in mind, though, that some medicines we use are poisonous to pets, and some of their meds are bad for us. Talk to your vet to find out options for your pet; I have a brief list in *Human Medicines that Are Safe for Dogs and Cats* on poly-species pharmacy.

Your minimum Pet Emergency Kit should have:

Documentation: copy of vaccination records and local registration
Shelter: a blanket, plus a crate or cage for them to travel and sleep in
Security: a leash and a collar, ideally with spare for each
Sustenance: 7 days supply of water *and* dry food (dry lasts longer & weighs less)
Morale: favorite chews and toys
Elimination: litter and litter box for cats; pooper-scooper and bags for dogs
Medications: flea collars, relevant prescription and OTC meds

DUAL-USE, OR EVEN MULTI-USE, SUPPLIES ARE A TREMENDOUS ASSET IN CASES OF disasters. On the other hand, I don't endorse using animal medications on humans, because of concerns over purity and other quality issues with medicines made for animals.

What about the opposite: Which human medications can be safely used on common household pets? For the most part, this will focus on over-the-counter medications.

For starters, remember what a smart Greek guy said a long time ago: It's the dose that makes the poison. Even the safest drug, if given in too large a dose, becomes toxic. Beyond that, make sure ALL medications are kept safe from pets and young children. I read one report of a large dog that had no problem prying off the tamper proof lid on a bottle of ibuprofen and chugging the syrupy orange flavored elixir. It almost killed him.

Next, let's list a few medicines that are safe in humans but **should NEVER be used in cats and/or dogs:**

Acetaminophen, also sold under trade names like Tylenol, Tempra, Feveral and Daytril, is highly toxic in cats and must not be used. Be aware that it is used as an ingredient in a lot of cough, cold and sleep medicines.

It may cause liver damage in dogs but is sometimes used in low doses for a short time under veterinary supervision.

Benzocaine (a topical anesthetic), the active ingredient in Lanacaine and several hemorrhoid preparations, causes a change in the chemical nature of hemoglobin, the oxygen carrier in blood, that can be a problem in high doses. Some sources say Anbesol is safe for use up to two times a day on your dog for mouth pain, but I think you would be wiser contacting your vet prior to using it.

Cannabis or any other street drug, even though getting kitty stoned may be pretty cute. Same goes for alcohol of any kind: ethanol, methanol, rubbing alcohol or ethylene glycol. The toxic dosage and other properties of these drugs are just not known well enough.

Coffee and tea that contain any significant amounts of caffeine. While not exactly drugs, caffeine, theobromine (a component found in chocolate) and theophylline are members of the class of drugs called Methylxanines. As every consumer of these products knows, they are central nervous system (CNS) and cardiovascular stimulants that in high doses can increase blood pressure (mild) and also cause nausea and vomiting.

Ibuprofen, sold under brand names including Motrin and Advil, should never be given to dogs. Drugs like ibuprofen and naproxen are the number one cause of pet poisonings, according to the 2007 report by the ASPCA Animal Poison Control Center. As little as a single pill can cause a stomach ulcer. Increasing doses will eventually cause kidney failure which, left untreated, will be fatal.

Inhalers like albuterol and other medications inhaled for control of asthma are not recommended, as they cause increased heart rate, excitement, restlessness, dizziness, nervousness or tremors.

Phenazopyridine, also known as pyridium and used in humans as a urinary analgesic and antiseptic, it causes red blood cell breakdown and liver injury in cats.

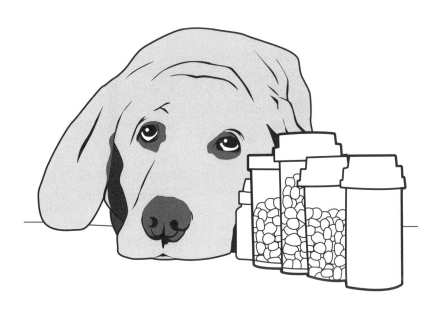

Phenytoin, used by humans for seizure control, is not recommended for use in dogs and cats as the drug levels are hard to predict and thus make the drug prone to toxicity, especially in cats.

Supplements, especially iron and Vitamins A and D, can be a problem the over long term. Pets are affected by chronic iron toxicity because they do not have a way to excrete excessive iron from their bodies.

Vitamins A and D are fat-soluble and can also accumulate to dangerous levels. Vitamin D can also cause sudden spikes in calcium levels in the blood and cause acute problems that way. Even though they are water soluble, vitamins B6 and C can also cause problems.

....

Now, let's move on to list a few drugs that can be safely used by cats and/or dogs, and their bipedal friends. Again, keep in mind that accurate dosing is just as important for pets as for us, often more so due to their small size. For this reason, liquid forms may be better since they can more easily be given in small amounts.

Antacids like Di-gel suspension (containing Aluminum/Magnesium/Simethicone) can be used to sooth an upset stomach in both cats and dogs.

Keep in mind that you run the risk of masking the symptoms of a serious condition at first, so it's best to consult your vet unless a true emergency forces you to make the call.

Anti-Diarrheal Agents, like Bismuth Subsalicylate (Pepto-Bismol) and Kaolin (Kaopectate) can be used as home remedies for doggy diarrhea. Again, the correct dosage depends on your dog's size, so use of children's formulations based on your dog's weight is best.

As with aspirin, another salicylate, Pepto-Bismol should not be used in felines, while Kaopectate is OK.

Aspirin, a drug most of us have on hand, has been meeting many human needs for many years prior to the use of Tylenol and Advil.

Like ibuprofen, aspirin belongs to the Non-Steroidal Anti-Inflammatory Drugs family, usually referred to as NSAIDs. NSAIDs are used to ease aches and pains, and also for reducing fevers. Aspirin is also used to reduce blood clots in humans. This is good news for some people, but usually not so for dogs.

Dogs are especially prone to NSAID-induced internal bleeding and ulcers if they get drugs like aspirin incorrectly. Because of this, aspirin usually should only be given under the direct supervision of your vet, who can tell you the proper dosage and interval between doses.

Common side effects of NSAIDs include vomiting, loss of appetite, depression, lethargy, and diarrhea. More dangerous side effects include gastrointestinal bleeding, stomach ulcers and perforation, kidney damage, and liver problems.

In most instances, you should use "baby" aspirin, and give it to your canine units with some food to help protect the lining of the stomach. Coated aspirin may offer some benefit as well.

Aspirin is *sometimes* used for cats, but only in very small doses and infrequently. Consult a vet first!!!!

Calamine lotion can be dabbed on itchy rashes and stings. Take care not to use too much or to put it where the animal may lick a lot off, as it contains zinc which can be toxic in high doses.

Dimenhydrinate, or Dramamine is not FDA approved, but it is commonly used in dogs and cats for both sedation and motion sickness relief, just as it is in those prone to travel troubles.

Diphenhydramine, or Benadryl, is useful for dogs and cats suffering from itch due to allergies as well as reactions to bee stings.

Epinephrine, in small doses, can be used for severe allergic reactions that result in shock or respiratory distress in pets.

Etodolac, sold to humans by prescription as Iodine, is one NSAID in addition to aspirin that is safe for both dogs and select non-pregnant humans. It is not known to be safe for cats.

Hydrocortisone cream or topical solutions offer relief for treating localized itching. After you apply these preparations, you should get the dog or cat involved in a fun activity, as pets tend to try licking the treated area.

These are poorly absorbed into the blood, and tend not create long-term side effects associated with oral or injectable steroids when used in moderation, up to twice a day to itchy areas.

Ketoprofen, sold to humans by prescription as orudis, is another NSAID besides aspirin that is safe for both dogs and cats, as well as some non-pregnant humans.

Mineral oil can be used as a laxative when given by mouth to both pets and humans. It should not be used in humans younger than about 6 years old or those who are debilitated or pregnant, or who have hiatal hernia, dysphagia, esophogeal or gastric retention. This is because of the risk of aspiration into the lungs.

To prevent aspiration in small animals, orally administered mineral oil should not be attempted when there is an increased risk of vomiting, regurgitation or other preexisting swallowing difficulty. Light mineral oil is also more risky than heavy forms with respect to aspiration,

Poisoning treatments like Hydrogen peroxide (which can be used to make a pet vomit) and Activated charcoal (used to absorb ingested poisons) can be helpful if your pet gets into something it shouldn't. Try to consult your veterinarian or the ASPCA Pet Poison Control Center before using.

Triple antibiotic ointment with neomycin, polymixin and bacitracin provides a broad spectrum of activity against many bacteria commonly involved in superficial infections of the skin. Apply up to four times daily on wounds to help prevent infection.

NOTE ···

As you can see, there is a wide range of medicines that you probably already have at home, and that you may be thinking about keeping on hand for bad times, that your four-legged family members may need, too. With good planning, plus input from your vet, or with close, careful work using the resources in the appendix for this chapter, you can safely use these multi-species meds!

Neighborhood and Community Analysis: Medical Threat Assessments

IN PLANNING FOR BAD TIMES, YOU MUST NOT NEGLECT TO CONSIDER YOUR LOCAL ENVIRONMENT: the neighborhood or community in which you live. This is true, like most of the other stuff in this book, whether or not you think we are in for a long, bad time due to economic collapse, energy descent or climate change. The things you learn when you perform a *medical threat assessment* (MTA) for your neighborhood (for those who live in a big city) or community will be valuable even if you never experience a disaster close to home.

Medical threat assessments look at environmental and other health-related factors that could have a negative impact on your daily activities by causing injury or disease, or by degrading your physical or mental performance.

The goal of these assessments is to be aware of, and prepared for, potential threats to your health. Examples of this might include having an adequate supply of safe water for hydration if you have to work outside in hot weather to clean up after a hurricane, or having a way to dispose of household wastes in the event of a disruption of garbage collection services.

Health comprises a huge array of factors including social, economic, emotional, environmental and physical inputs. Because of this, just about anything in your life could be considered an element to be included in a medical threat assessment. For the purposes of this book, however, I'm limiting the idea of threat to physical causes of disease.

A useful model for this is the *epidemiologic triad* of host—agent—environment. Basically this means that an *agent* exists or acts through the *environment* to cause disease in a *host*, meaning you, your family members or other persons, or an animal such as a pet. Your goal in a medical threat assessment is thus to understand those factors that exist in the environment that could allow agents like infectious pathogens or environmental poisons to cause disease. Malaria is a classic example of the triad: A swampy environment allows mosquitoes to breed and spread the malaria agent to human hosts. There may also be medical factors you or those close to you have that you should consider in these assessments.

Perhaps the first step in completing any MTA is to define your population at risk or PAR: For whom are you doing this assessment? For most of us, the PAR would comprise ourselves, plus in all likelihood our family and friends. Once you define the PAR, or *who*, ask yourself questions such as *where, what* and *when*? These are the main things you need to consider in your MTA. Once you've established the who, you need to obtain some other basic information about the situation to answer the where, what and when questions.

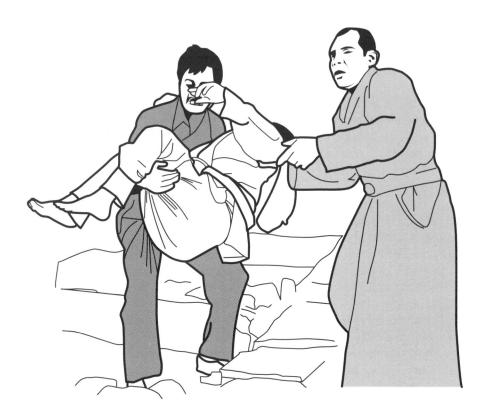

Another facet of the *who* question has to do with who lives near you. Do you have a strong neighborhood association or other group that gives cohesiveness to those who live around you? Regardless, you should learn about your neighbors. Who could help with rescue and medical aid after an earthquake? Who would be likely to need rescue? After a disaster, the pastor who lives up the street may be a great ally for psychological first aid efforts, for example.

Where implies the geography, terrain, climate and weather patterns of the place you live. Companies, NGOs and military organizations focus on planning for the places they will be working, their *area of operations*. For disaster planning, and getting ready for gridcrash or other infrastructure collapses, you should formulate plans based on your area of operations, that is, the area where you live, work and otherwise travel frequently.

Threats to your health will be different when you move from the cool, dry mountains of the West to the hot, sticky Southeast. Some communities have weather patterns that make severe storms a yearly event, while others may lie on an active earthquake fault. Your risks for environmental injuries due to altitude, radiation, plants and animals are all related in part to where you live. The point is that you should get to know your physical environment.

We live in an information age, but it's important to consider that with the explosion of information comes the concern that some information may not be reliable.

Perhaps the most reliable source of information is history. Part of the reason we worry about disasters is because they have occurred in the past, so we know they will occur in the future.

For starters, look back at the recent history of weather and geologic events in your area. You should know if blizzards, droughts, flooding, heat waves, hurricanes and/or tornadoes have been frequent occurrences. Other potential threats to note may include wild fires, landslides or earthquakes.

Next you should know if there are poisonous animals such as scorpions or snakes native to your area. Find out before you have to go rooting around in the bush where they will be hiding. Check to find out if there are problems with large predatory mammals. Recent mountain lion attacks in the West highlight the importance of this consideration.

In addition, you should know if there are hazardous plants such as poison ivy in your area. It might also be important to know if any of your houseplants or the plants in your garden are poisonous to humans or animals, especially if you have kids or pets.

Look at these issues applied to the areas that you travel to and visit frequently and where you work as well. In addition, you should have an idea of industries in your area and potential hazards they portend. It would be useful to know, for instance, if the railroad line about a quarter mile from your house carries train cars containing chlorine gas or other potential hazards in the event of derailment, either accidental or caused by intentional action due to terrorism or crime.

Your local fire department, public health department or environmental health or quality department at the state level may know this information. Some states or cities publish information like this in their disaster plans.

In terms of *what,* you should think about both human factors and environmental factors that will impact on agents that cause disease as well as *vectors* that help disease transmission.

Military and police planners as well as nongovernmental organizations that do business overseas have to think about "battle injuries" as a major concern in their threat assessments. Intentional injuries like homicide and suicide must also be considered. While crime and terrorism could potentially cause these types of injuries here at home, I won't talk much about them as part of an MTA. I will, however, address security issues in the chapter on ethics when there is no doctor.

Most of the *what* has to do with injuries from machinery, sports, falls, transportation accidents and other events of daily life that are major causes of death and disability in modern society. Think about how you and your loved ones can mitigate these risks; I recognize that life is not without risk. The philosophy behind medical threat assessments is limitation, not elimination, of exposure to risk.

In situations of conflict and catastrophe, infectious disease has been shown time and time again to be the major threat to public health. Consider, for example, that measles outbreaks in refugee camps are major killers, or that cholera sickened 200,000 people and killed 12,000 after the civil war in Rwanda in the '90s, making the suffering from the war itself that much worse. Poor hygiene, close contact among humans or between human beings and animals, as well as host factors like fatigue and malnutrition all increase susceptibility to disease in these settings.

We talked in the last chapter about the importance of psychological stress inoculation and psychological first aid to help prevent and treat the psychological injury that can occur in disasters. In this context, think also about special populations such as children and how you can prepare them in advance for the major disaster threats in your area, thereby saving them some of the distress they might otherwise feel when they occur.

Finally, when thinking about *when,* think not only about threats that occur during times when infrastructure is normal, but also when infrastructure is distinctly abnormal. Think about how natural disaster, civil strife, economic collapse or energy crisis will affect the areas you live, work and play in.

Prioritizing this list of threats will be a huge task. By focusing on the biggest potential threats, you will be more likely to actually get something done, rather than spending your whole time on the plan. Consider using a 2 x 2 matrix like the one shown in the figure combining likelihood and severity of events.. It is most beneficial to spend your time, effort and money in developing countermeasures to those threats in quadrant I, because they have the highest combined likelihood and severity.

An alternative to the medical threat analysis model, the *SWOT* matrix, has been used by business schools and other management programs for years. You look at the Strengths and Weaknesses as well as the Opportunities and Threats for your organization.

A SWOT analysis for your area should consider all the things you and your family need for sustainability. Think imaginatively: Can you get water, food, shelter, security, energy, waste disposal, transportation and entertainment needs met via local resources, even if they are not the usual way of doing things? You may have resources you are not aware of or that you don't acknowledge are there because you take them for granted.

Is there a body of water you could use to collect and purify water for your family nearby? Woods where you could collect deadfall for firewood as an emergency source of fuel for cooking, light and heat? You may have other assets like locally grown food, strong public mass transit or any number of other factors; keep an open mind.

In terms of weaknesses, you may notice that some of the items listed above are not available. Maybe you live in the concrete jungle where growing food on a large scale is not possible. You may not be able to change that, but you can look at options like having a few days' worth of food on hand rather than stopping at the Kwik-E-Mart or neighborhood grocery every day for your food. Maybe you have a balcony and can grow some staples like potatoes, tomatoes and the like in pots.

As you review the strengths and weaknesses of your area, look for other opportunities, like a neighborhood or community garden. In terms of opportunities related to health knowledge, skills and behaviors in your neighborhood or community, think expansively. You may find that you live near a school where you can learn valuable health and hygiene skills. Maybe your county public health department will help you get free vaccinations or provide other preventive health measures at low cost, helping you to maximize your health prior to gridcrash.

Threats will generally be the geological and weather-related issues that we talked about above, plus things that move through your area on roads or rail, or are stored near your home. Other threats may be poor sanitation or environmental quality. With a failed infrastructure comes a breakdown of normal safeguards, making these threats potentially more dangerous to you. It pays to keep a wary eye on them.

....

Conclusion:

Regardless of whether you use a medical threat analysis framework or the SWOT matrix, the logistical planning you do now can go a long way towards protecting your health in the event of gridcrash, well before you need medical help or expertise. Keep in mind that human beings are essentially living machines, and medical threat assessment allows us to plan for preventive maintenance on our human machinery during gridcrash or other disaster. Activities that you continue after the crash can have a positive impact on your health, including a lot of things we've talked about already in terms of morale and discipline, as well as rest and hydration. In the next chapter, we'll talk about hygiene and sanitation as well as protective equipment that will help limit the incidence of injuries as well as infectious diseases.

Suggested First Aid Kit Items

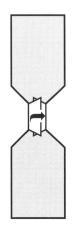

- First Aid Handbook
- Durable container: plastic box most common
- Personal Protective Equipment (PPE)
- Disposable Gloves, non-sterile, several pairs, nitrile (avoid latex due to allergies)
- Goggles or spray shield to cover eyes
- CPR mask (or other barrier such as a face shield)
- Alcohol rub (hand sanitizer) or antiseptic hand wipes
- Sunscreen
- Access to Patient
- Trauma shears (for cutting clothing, bandages, etc.)
- Flashlight
- Patient Assessment tools
- Thermometer
- Penlight
- Wound Care: scrapes, cuts and burns
  - Shur-Clens or other non-ionic wound prep
  - Saline for irrigation
  - Dressings (to be applied directly to wound, so must be sterile)
  - Absorbent compress 5"x9" (ABD pad)
  - 2"x2" and 4"x4" Gauze Pads
  - Non-adherent pads (like Telfa)
  - Burn dressings (commercial purpose-made)
  - Occlusive dressings like Vaseline Gauze
  - Bandages (non-sterile, primarily to secure a dressing)
  - Gauze roller bandages, 2" and 4" (like Kerlix or Kling)
  - Elastic bandages (for pressure dressing)
  - Triangular bandages (2-3 for slings, tying splints, many other uses)
  - Adhesive bandages
  - Straight adhesive bandages like Band Aids
  - Butterfly (knuckle) bandages
  - Adhesive tape, hypoallergenic
  - Self-adherent bandage like Coban
  - Antibiotic ointment: single, double or triple
  - Cotton balls (for applying ointments, creams)
  - Tweezers (for splinter or tick removal)
- Sprain/Strain/Fracture Care Equipment
  - Splints for immobilization

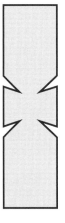

Sticky side (shown in gray)

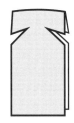

- SAM Splint (malleable aluminum padded with foam)
- Wire ladder splint
- Tongue blades or other finger splints (two)
- CE or similar elastic bandages (see above)
- Chemical cold packs (break and shake instant cold)
- Safety pins for making slings, etc. (Assorted sizes)
■ Eye Injury Care Supplies
  - Eye cup or small plastic cup
  - Sterile eye pads
  - Sterile eye wash (saline packaged for contact lenses)
■ Patient Protection
  - Emergency "space blanket" (lightweight plastic foil blankets)
■ Medications
  - See list above of OTC medications for home storage for suggestions
  - (Small, single use packets are best for FAKs due to convenience)
■ Hemorrhage Control (see *Stop the Bleeding!*)
  - Tourniquet
  - Hemostatic agents like Celox or QuikClot
■ Amputation preservation kit (1 large garbage bag, 4 kitchen-sized & 2 bread bags)
■ Saran wrap and tampons (see *Household Items for First Aid*)
■ A few dollars worth of quarters secured in the box
(for emergency phone calls)

Stop the Bleeding!   TIP

BLEEDING IS A COMMON RESULT OF MANY OF THE DAY-TO-DAY INJURIES WE SUSTAIN, from scrapes, cuts and the like. Treating bleeding is also a major focus of most basic first aid courses. Sometimes bleeding can be severe enough that it becomes life-threatening. In these situations, control of bleeding can truly be lifesaving.

Hemorrhage control is also a subject of controversy. The tourniquet, traditionally taught as a tool of last resort, has seen a bit of a comeback lately due to successful use in military medical care. Some have advocated that it should be used more frequently in civilian care as well. Others have likened it to the Devil's pitchfork.

There are a number of alternatives to tourniquets that probably will work for more than 95% of bleeding events. A compression dressing, created with a big wad of gauze on top of the wound wrapped with a tight elastic bandage to squeeze things down, works most of the time. There are some specialized dressings that allow you to create this effect in a smaller package, but at higher cost and with less flexibility. You can also use the ACE-type bandage to wrap a sprain, secure a splint or sling an arm. It's hard to do that with the specialty bandages designed for hemorrhage control.

Another recent development in hemorrhage control is the hemostatic agent. Agents like Celox and HemCon can be poured or placed into a bleeding wound to help clot blood and thus stop the flow. These agents have had some kinks that are being worked out. They are expensive, too, and can't be cleaned and re-used like a tourniquet.

Current Red Cross and other first-aid guidelines recommend against tourniquet use, but I think that you should consider them if your circumstance routinely puts you at high risk for severe bleeding. Who do I include in this group? I would say if there is a chance you could be shot by a high-powered weapon (hunters and Law Enforcement Officers, for example) or suffer an amputated or crushed limb (farmers, loggers or deep sea fishermen come to mind) that you should become familiar with proper techniques for tourniquet use and that you have one available in case you need to save a coworker's life, or your own. ●

CHAPTER 4

Preventive Medicine

Preventive Medicine:
Protecting Health When There Is No Doctor

LIFE, THOMAS HOBBES FAMOUSLY WROTE, CAN BE "NASTY, BRUTISH, AND SHORT." IN LARGE part it was all of these things because of disease, which prior to the Industrial Revolution was usually attributed to mystical powers. The word influenza, after all, comes from Italian for the concept of a person being influenced by bad spirits.

We now have the benefit of a more complete, concrete understanding of disease, particularly due to the host-agent-environment model we talked about in the last chapter. In this regard, we are ahead of our predecessors. In other ways, though, they had an advantage over us because they didn't have a huge technological arsenal on which they could rely for help in fighting disease.

In a sense, the collapse of modern medical infrastructure will send us full-circle. We will have to learn be especially vigilant in our efforts to stay healthy and prevent disease, because some curative measures may not be readily available anymore. Drugs and medical supplies we now use daily may be hard to come by. Luckily, we can combine our current knowledge with the best of what came before to improve our situation when it comes to health, no matter how far down the slippery slope we slide.

This chapter will focus on some of the many things we can learn from the days before medicine embraced the technological imperative: What simple preventive measures can we practice like good hygiene, sunlight and fresh air to lessen the burden of infectious disease? How do we reduce injury, that other old nemesis? Finally, how can we maximize non-pharmacologic strategies to deal with potentially debilitating diseases without modern artificially made drugs?

Infection Control

WE KNOW THAT PRIOR TO MODERN, INDUSTRIALIZED MEDICINE AND ITS IMPRESSIVE ARRAY OF surgical saves and antibiotic choices, most people died from injury or infection. The *epidemiologic transition* took us away from those killers, with the tradeoff that we now survive, only to die later, in most cases from heart disease, cancer or stroke. This transition has now reached most of the world, even the poorer societies of the southern tier of the world's countries.

Now, while we still worry about infectious disease, the days of fearing for our children in the summer because of polio and in the winter because of influenza are largely behind us.

Hubris is dangerous, however, and we have paid for our medical hubris in the past few years: SARS, HIV/AIDS, multi-drug resistant superbugs like MRSA and resurgent diseases like tuberculosis all point out the danger of letting down our guard by thinking we had infections licked.

In a time of epidemic disease, like pandemic flu, or after some form of societal collapse, we may face a reversal of the epidemiologic transition. Infection may again become a big deal, not just something we fight off with a quick dose of the latest oral antibiotic.

When these hard times hit, infection control measures that are cheap, easy and low-tech, will be a better bet than high-tech solutions. Most experts admit that there won't be enough vaccine or anti-viral medicines available fast enough to help everyone in the face of a severe flu pandemic like the one the world experienced in 1918, or if avian influenza becomes easily spread among humans.

Even if there were enough of these agents, we know that vaccines don't always work. Neither do medicines. In December of 2008, the CDC published guidance on the use of medications for influenza during flu season. It was issued in response to data from some states showing that a large proportion of the influenza viruses found there were resistant to the influenza-specific antiviral medication oseltamivir (Tamiflu). This is not surprising, as worldwide the number of flu viruses that show resistance to Tamiflu has been increasing. Other infectious agents like SARS don't yet have effective medical treatments.

In light of this, infection control measures offer some hope: Influenza epidemics often occur in waves. If you avoid infection in the first wave, you may have a less severe infection if you get sick in a later wave, or there may be new vaccines or medicines available for you by the time you do get sick.

What are some of the measures that we can take now, in our everyday lives, and later, in the event of a bigger threat? We will talk about a few ways that have been shown to decrease infection that won't require much effort but could offer big rewards, and others that may take more time, planning and expenditure, but may be critical.

A Show of Hands, Please

THE FIRST, MOST IMPORTANT COMMANDMENT OF INFECTION CONTROL IS *WASH YOUR HANDS*. Early and often! How often? Studies on infectious viruses like flu and the common cold have shown that hand washing at least ten times per day helps reduce the occurrence of infection by 55% *without any other interventions*.

This is because most respiratory infections and others, like a lot of GI bugs, are transmitted by contact: You touch a germ-laden surface, then you touch a portal of entry into your body or someone else's. The eyes, nose and mouth are most commonly the portal; think how many times you touch these areas as you go through your day, usually without even knowing you're doing it.

It may seem silly to ask, really, but exactly how do you wash your hands? No fancy disinfectants needed: just soap, water and friction. Studies in hospitals show that the tips of the fingers are frequently missed while the palms and backs of the hand get too much time. Long fingernails hide a lot of germs; keep nails short (< 5mm of "nail length" beyond the bed, according to the WHO) if you are worried about hygiene. A good lather, with vigorous friction for about 30-60 seconds followed by a rinse with clean, preferably warm, water suffices.

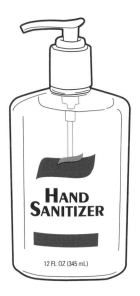

In the OR, we use either foot pedals to control the flow of water, or use our elbows to turn off the tap. This way, we don't have to worry about recontaminating our hands. You can either wash the knobs for the faucet with the soapy lather while you wash your hands, or just shut off the flow by holding a clean paper towel in you hand. In the same way, be careful that you don't pick up any contamination from the doorknob on your way out of the washroom.

Alcohol-based waterless hand sanitizers are great if your hands aren't visibly soiled, and they are easily carried in convenient pocket-sized bottles if you are on the go. Just make sure you use them properly. You should also avoid using this "hand goo" too many times in a row, as the moisturizers and other chemicals in the gels will build up on your hands; just wash with soap and water in between to remove the leftover gunk.

As important as hand washing is, too much can actually make things worse. Soap can dry skin and make it more susceptible to infection, and frequent washing can also change the makeup of the bugs that live on hands.

Despite this, good hand hygiene helps prevent infection with a variety of organisms. The bugs can go in either direction: You can get them from others, or they can get them from you. Infection can come from respiratory ailments like the flu, common cold, SARS and chickenpox, or gastrointestinal goodies like diarrheal illnesses. The latter are spread by so-called fecal-oral route—ponder, for a few seconds, what that means!

An Austro-Hungarian obstetrician named Ignaz Semmelweis noted about 150 years ago that doctors, who were doing autopsies barehanded prior to delivering babies, struggled with high rates of maternal childbed fever afflicting their patients. He also observed that midwives, who didn't do autopsies, had no such troubles. He made the doctors start washing their hands with a bleach solution after autopsies, et voila!, the rates of childbed fever equalized. Since then, we have known what to do, but alas, we don't always do what we know.

We know, for example, that most members of the public don't wash their hands frequently enough, and when they do wash, they don't do so for long enough.

You don't need antibiotic or antiseptic ingredients, which have been shown to foster bacterial resistance. Instead, wash frequently with soap and warm water (hot water can damage skin) if your skin is grossly soiled, but otherwise try to use alcohol-based hand sanitizer with a moisturizer. The alcohol will kill bacteria, viruses and fungi, and won't dry your skin too much.

In some special circumstances, you may consider using a soap with antibacterial properties rather than regular soap; see the table.

Reasons You May Need Antibacterial Soap

- If you have close physical contact with persons at high risk for infection (e.g., neonates, the very old, or immunosuppressed).
- If you have close physical contact with infected persons; infection with an organism likely to be transmitted by direct contact (diarrhea, upper respiratory infection, skin infections).
- Or if you work in a setting in which infectious disease transmission is likely (food preparation, crowded living quarters such as chronic-care residences, prisons, child-care centers, and preschools)

Hot Hand, Cold Hand

TWENTY YEARS AGO OR SO, I WORKED IN A RESEARCH LAB AS AN UNDERGRAD AT THE UNIVERSITY of Washington. I handled radioactive materials as part of my work, and learned a few techniques from the radiation safety officers there that I carry with me today. The key is the "hot hand, cold hand" technique.

Hot obviously refers to radiation, but now I label the hot hand as the one touching stuff I don't want to spread: It may be the hand doing the wiping of baby's bottom with the diaper wipe. I use just one hand for the dirty tasks, and reserve the other hand (held behind the back as a reminder if need be), which is uncontaminated, for touching common-use items until I can wash both hands.

Bear in mind that contamination on gloves can spread to clean areas, and although you may remain protected, others could be exposed if you are careless. If there is potential for contamination of your gloves, you must remove your gloves before handling common-use items.

Remove gloves by turning them inside out. Grab the outside surface of one glove with the other, gloved hand. Strip the glove off, allowing it to turn inside out. Don't ever insert gloved fingers inside a glove to assist in removal. Once the first glove is off, the fingers of the ungloved hand can be inserted inside the second glove to affect its removal. Do not blow into gloves to try to restore them to their original shape for repeat use as this allows opportunity for ingestion of material from a dirty glove.

Finally, as we talked about in a previous chapter, plastic bags or wrap can be used as impromptu gloves or protective clothing in an emergency, but you should avoid routine use of this technique.

Don't Be Coughy

THE CDC RECOMMENDS THE FOLLOWING COUGH ETIQUETTE MEASURES TO LIMIT THE SPREAD of infectious respiratory secretions of individuals who have symptoms of a respiratory infection, in addition to good hand-washing.

- ■ Cover your nose and mouth when coughing or sneezing; it's best to cover with a tissue, handkerchief or your sleeve if need be.
- ■ Use tissues to contain respiratory secretions, and dispose of them in the nearest waste receptacle after use.
- ■ Carry alcohol-based hand rub for times when sinks aren't available for hand-washing.

Protect Yourself

PERSONAL PROTECTIVE EQUIPMENT, OR PPE, HAS ALSO BEEN SHOWN TO HELP REDUCE disease transmission. Again, simple measures suffice. You don't need a full spaceman biohazard suit like Dustin Hoffman wore in the movie *Outbreak*, just cheap things like masks and gloves.

Taken together, a mask, gloves, gown and hand washing will help reduce your odds of infection from viral respiratory illnesses like the cold, influenza and maybe even SARS by over 90%! Most of the protective effect of PPE seems to come from masks (and hand washing) while gowns and gloves are most useful if you are dealing with bodily fluids, for instance taking care of ill infants or debilitated people.

Obviously you need to have these supplies on hand in advance, as you learned last chapter in the discussion about planning a sickroom. Most of these items are disposable, but in a pinch many can be re-used with proper care.

Gloves should be used once and thrown away, unless you have to resort to heavier dishwashing gloves, which could be washed and treated with bleach then dried for re-use.

Gowns, either disposable plastic or reusable cloth surgical gowns, are probably not needed unless you are dealing with a sick person's bodily fluids.

When it comes to masks, most of us are familiar with painter's masks and similar masks used in the OR. They are designed to catch large droplets, but offer only minimal protection against smaller particles like viruses, bacteria and spores that we could inhale to cause disease. Because of this, the CDC, WHO and OSHA, among others, recommend that all employees entering a patient care area where airborne transmission of infection is possible use a Filtering Facepiece Respirator, or FFR, like an N95, N99 or N100 mask.

What exactly is the difference between an FFR and a surgical mask? Surgical masks can provide some protection against larger droplets that are considered to be the primary route of some infectious disease transmission, but don't effectively protect against some particles, because they allow for leakage through or around the mask. FFRs, when properly fitted, provide an adequate barrier against both large and small aerosolized droplets that may be encountered.

Ideally you should only use the FFR for which you have been "fit tested." If you can find an occupational medicine center or similar facility in your area, or where you work, I highly recommend that you have a respirator fit testing session to help you pick and size a respirator. Some people say you can try testing the mask for leaks yourself, but I think this is dicey, especially for serious infections.

During SARS, we saw pictures of people on trains or walking in the street wearing face masks, a repeat of the cloth masks on policemen in the US in some pictures from the 1918 "Spanish Flu" outbreak. There is some data that show you can use similarly fashioned cloth masks, although these are not ideal.

Improvised mask: Researchers simply boiled a Hanes Heavyweight 100% preshrunk cotton T-shirt for 10 minutes to maximize shrinkage and sterilize the material, then air-dried it. Next, they cut out an outer layer for tying on the mask and filled it with 8 inner layers. While not perfect, it did offer one person who tested it 67% of the protection of a perfectly fitted commercial N95 mask.

Finally, remember that FFRs are designed to be disposable after being used once. You may run out, though, in a pandemic. Most makers of the masks are running low on supply as folks in hospitals and the government race to stockpile PPE. We saw a run on these masks during the early swine flu experience here.

During SARS in Taiwan, the cost of these masks went up by a factor of 20 or so. If you follow the recommendations of the Institute of Medicine you might be able to safely re-use FFRs: Obviously the mask shouldn't be soiled, torn, or creased. Wearing a surgical mask over the FFR, and keeping the FFR stored so it is safe from contamination or damage (by getting wet or crushed) may help. Wash your hands before putting it on or removing it. There is currently no approved method to decontaminate these masks, although theoretically sun could help. (See below.)

Let the Sun Shine

HELIOTHERAPY, OR USE OF LIGHT FROM THE SUN FOR THERAPEUTIC PURPOSES, HAS A RICH tradition in medicine that has largely been replaced by concern about the risk of skin cancer and other skin diseases from sun exposure.

Around WWI, a Swiss physician named Oskar Bernhard was treating a soldier with a complex wound infection from surgery for a gunshot wound. He remembered "mountain peasants" in his alpine homeland using a technique of drying meat in sun to preserve it and keep it from rotting. This doctor moved the patient into the sun, where he lay with his wound covered with light gauze; miraculously, his wound began to heal.

Another use of sunlight was for the treatment of Tuberculosis, or TB. TB was a common killer before the antibiotic era, and beyond affecting the lungs also infected bones and other tissues, which were often treated with deforming surgeries. Some physicians noted that gradually longer sunbaths seemed to help those with TB, especially TB of the bones. The TB asylum, with its open

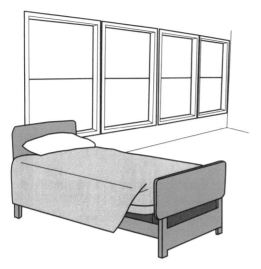

porches crowded with patients in the sun, is another historical oddity making a comeback.

The key component of sunlight when it comes to infection is ultraviolet radiation, or UV. UV can cause mutations in DNA that result in the death of bacteria and viruses; unfortunately in animals like us, UV-induced mutations can also lead to development of cancers like melanoma.

UV light has three bands, and the UV-C band is the most effective at killing infectious organisms. UV-B can also work, but is less efficient. Sunlight has very little UV-C, so it takes longer for natural sun to work its magic.

Many hospitals and clinics use artificial UV-C lights to help prevent infection, mounted above eye level and directed upward to help sanitize air as it circulates without causing problems for humans. Air circulates within these rooms, so particles of dust (and dead skin cells) acting as "rafts" for germs are exposed to the light as they float around the room. This helps reduce infection risks.

So there was a reason beyond a cheery atmosphere that I told you that your sickroom should be made open to the sun. You might even consider adding a UV-C light of your own to the sickroom, or the area just outside it, to bolster the effects of the sun's rays.

A Breath of Fresh Air

ANOTHER OLDER BUT STILL USEFUL TECHNIQUE FOR FIGHTING INFECTION IS VENTILATION. Toxicologists, the medical specialists who treat overdoses and other poisonings, often quip that "when it comes to pollution, dilution is the solution!" This solution can also be applied to infection.

Some infections can be transmitted via the airborne route: They can travel a long distance from the source patient to the next recipient. Others, like influenza, require passage on larger droplets that don't move through the air very well. In either case, though, keeping air moving is helpful.

Modern hospitals take advantage of these facts by using ventilation to help reduce infection. Rooms are required to have a certain number of air changes per hour (ACH). One ACH means that the air in a room is completely replaced by air from a different source each hour. Unfortunately, modern buildings are sealed up tight, and about 2/3 or more of the new air simply comes from somewhere else in the building.

Obviously this can lead to problems if there is a potential source of infection in the building. One study of a nursing home consisting of four different buildings showed how this matters: One building that had no recirculated air had a much lower number of flu cases during one outbreak than the other three buildings, which recirculated 30–70% of their air.

Taking this a bit further, researchers in Peru showed that older hospitals, with big, open windows and high ceilings, had much more efficient air circulation than modern hospitals with isolation rooms built specifically to recirculate the air. In models of TB spread, the open wards worked better than modern designs at protecting patients and staff from risk of acquiring TB from a source patient. No need for gale-force winds, either—a breeze of just 2 km/h (only 1.2 mph) was enough to offer protection. The isolation rooms actually had fewer ACH than their design specifications promised due to poor maintenance.

Keeping your house light and airy, then, probably helps reduce the risk to the occupants for infection. Other design features that reduce infection transmission risk include having as much space per person as possible within residential buildings. Many of these measures are being applied in resource poor areas of the world, as simple seems to be better. In hard times, these measures could be applied to "rich" parts of the world with similar success.

Keep to Yourself

IN ANY SEVERE EPIDEMIC, AUTHORITIES MAY INSTITUTE SOCIAL DISTANCING MEASURES LIKE canceling school, church, sports and other mass gatherings in hopes of stopping or at least slowing the epidemic. The utility of these measures in past epidemics like the 1918 flu outbreak or the recent SARS epidemic is hotly debated in the public health profession. You should, however, anticipate that these measures will be instituted despite this controversy: They are part of current plans. I think it pays to heed them, at least until you know they don't help.

I say this because there were some so-called *escape communities* during the 1918 flu pandemic that experienced dramatically lower rates of death and disease by closing their gates, canceling meetings or otherwise implementing social distancing measures. The choice, as always, is entirely yours, but I think it is important that you know about this issue.

Whaddya Gonna Do with All That Junk?

A CRUCIAL DETERMINANT OF HEALTH IS WASTE MANAGEMENT. KEEP IN MIND THAT THE AVERAGE adult produces 10 pounds of waste per day. In the West, and many parts of the developing world, we take waste disposal for granted. Keep in mind, though, that one of the reasons we don't live in a medical Hobbesian nightmare is that we have access to a marvelous system of plumbing that brings us clean water and whisks away our waste. We can recycle or dispose of our non-human waste easily, too, although in some rural areas that may mean taking it to the landfill ourselves.

One thing we have seen before is the effect of flooding on sewers and drinking water supplies: Summers around where I live often are sprinkled with warnings to boil water before drinking it or using it for hygienic measures. City dwellers also understand why strikes by trash collectors often seem to occur in the summer, when pressure to end them rises with the stench of the uncollected curbside debris.

Some waste will harbor infectious organisms that can spread throughout your household or community. Waste also attracts insects and vermin that can easily act as vectors of disease. It harms morale and quality of life, too, because of smell, flies, and other unpleasant physical qualities. All of these considerations demand that you have some way of dealing with waste. Reduce, reuse, repurpose and recycle can be applied to some forms of waste, but biological (human and animal) waste requires special considerations.

Your planning measures can exert a profound impact here: Remember that in addition to food, water and medicine, you should have enough materials for good sanitation on hand. In the event of a longer term problem, you may need to be able to bury or burn waste. See the tip *Waste at the End of the World* for a suggested list of sanitation and hygiene supplies to have handy.

TIP ▸ Waste at the End of the World

WASTE MANAGEMENT WILL BECOME A HUGE ISSUE DURING ANY MAJOR DISRUPTION of societal infrastructure. Current models predict that at least 40% of the workforce will not show up in event of a flu pandemic. Picture what this means, having only two thirds of the waste collection you have now. How many times do you take full garbage cans to the curb for the weekly pickup; what if you had to wait another week for pickup?

We know the average produce person produces roughly 10 pounds of total waste per day. In terms of stinky stuff, it is estimated that the average person produces somewhere around 140 pounds of excreta per year, or about ½ pound per day. This all has to go somewhere. If it doesn't get handled properly, filth and smell will be only one of the problems. Disease is a much more serious concern, as we know from outbreaks of diarrheal diseases, which are among the leading causes of childhood death in the Third World.

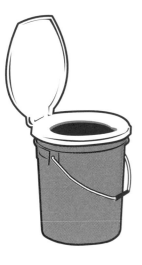

Although somewhat indelicate, this discussion obviously has to take place. How can you deal with the human waste produced in the event flush toilets aren't available? In part, how we deal with disruptions will depend on the length of time of interruption of basic services that you can expect to have to put up with after a disaster. If things are going to be back online relatively soon, you may choose the bucket method.

In this method, solid waste is deposited in a large bucket (like a 5 Gallon plastic bucket; you can even buy toilet seats to fit these!) then covered with something like sawdust, ashes, kitty litter or diatomaceous earth to cut down on pests and odor. This expedient toilet is stored in a part of your dwelling where it will be out of the way, ideally outside of living areas, such as on the patio, in a garage or in a corner of the lawn.

If things are expected to be bad for longer, you can use improvised latrines provided you can keep them safe from the water supply. Everybody who's been through scouting and earned the Camping merit badge knows how to dig a simple latrine. Dig latrines deep but above the water table, so that animals don't dig them up and the water won't be contaminated. Any latrine should be at least 200 yards from a water source, ideally downhill. Obviously you need a shovel and perhaps a pick in order to be able to dig a latrine; you may not currently have these, so if you have plans to build a latrine in an emergency, make sure you acquire the tools in advance of need.

More complex latrine designs can also be dug in the event things get really bad for a long time. For more information on design and construction of latrines, see the discussion of prison hygiene as a model for health at the end of the world in the next chapter.

Food waste such as scraps are also potential sources not only of unpleasant odors, but are also food sources for vermin such as rats, raccoons and stray pets. Ideally, you should separate refuse into compostable and non-compostable materials. Food waste can be used again, either as food for domestic animals or for compost.

Non-compostable materials (including paper or plastic are slower to break down, so these as well as medical waste from dressing and the like should probably be stored safely for later collection short-term. If waste collection will be interrupted for a prolonged period of time, this waste should be burned in an incinerator.

As part of your planning and preparation, you might consider having a store of the following items needed to help keep things clean. Note that a lot of these items are on the sickroom list:

■ 5 Gallon buckets (used, but clean, for use as emergency toilets)
■ Sawdust, kitty litter or diatomaceous earth (for covering waste in bucket)
■ Toilet Paper
■ Bleach (unscented, plain bleach and lots of it)
■ Air Freshener or deodorizer spray
■ Garbage bags
■ Laundry Detergent
■ Paper Towels
■ Cleaning Supplies
■ Bleach wipes
■ Sprays like Lysol or Formula 409
■ Dish or other liquid soap
■ Sponges and scrubbing pads
■ Vinegar
■ Baking soda
■ Feminine Napkins/Tampons
■ Lady-J or similar device (allows females to stand while urinating)
■ Shampoo and Conditioner
■ Bar Soaps (3-4 ounces per person each month)
■ Hand Sanitizers
■ Deodorant
■ Toothpaste and tooth brushes

- Dental floss
- Hand and body lotions
- Facial tissues (Kleenex, etc.)
- Diapers and wipes (age appropriate, as needed)
- Razors and shaving cream, soap or gel

Keep in mind that the things that we throw away or otherwise leave behind are a potential goldmine as potential resources when "repurposed" to another use. Even something as simple as 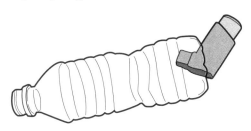 burning waste paper to generate heat in the winter or to use for cooking must not be overlooked. In the health care realm, the lowly plastic water bottle, for example, has a number of uses potentially including making insect traps, purifying water using the UV light of the sun, or making air chambers to increase the effectiveness of inhaled medicines for asthma and emphysema. The inside surfaces of sterile bandage wrappers or IV fluid bags can be used as occlusive dressings. In very austere circumstances, your trash could be converted to your treasure with some imagination and creativity.

Taken together, your efforts at waste disposal that are undertaken both before and after the onset of hard times will help to keep you healthy, safe and comfortable regardless of the situation.

Bring Out Your Dead!

AN UNAVOIDABLE SUBJECT FOR A BOOK LIKE THIS IS DEATH. OBVIOUSLY MY AIM IN THIS collection of measures for protecting health is ultimately to reduce the risk of death, but in a natural disaster like the recent Haiti quake or other major events, we will see large numbers of dead people. In case the authorities are overwhelmed, we need to know the basics for dealing with human remains, ideally in a non-Pythonesque manner!

I won't talk about the forensic aspects here, and will assume you will use this knowledge only in the event of a true emergency, just as you would not practice medicine without a license unless things are really dire. You should anticipate that if things do fall apart, you might be expected to justify how you handled this situation once normalcy returns.

First, even though the division of labor inherent to modern society may dissolve after hard times are here again, you should ideally delegate the task of handling dead bodies to a few select persons. This will protect the psyche of some, and the physical health of others, not chosen to do these tasks.

Next, don't neglect the needs of the living when you are dealing with the dead. Never put other lives at risk to recover or dispose of the dead; there may be some victims trapped in rubble or in other situations where you won't be able to get to them safely. Don't add to the death toll needlessly.

Finally, keep in mind that dead bodies from natural disasters don't cause epidemics; the living play a much greater role in spreading disease. Bodies can cause disease if their feces, which leaks after death, contaminates water used by the living.

On the other hand, bodies during epidemics may transmit disease if the dead are infected. See *Management of Dead Bodies in A Disaster* for other information.

TIP   ## Management of Dead Bodies in a Disaster

HOW DO YOU DEAL WITH THE BODIES OF DISASTER VICTIMS? THE PAN-AMERICAN Health Organization (PAHO) published a guide called *The Management of Dead Bodies after Disasters: A Field Guide for First Responders*. It can be downloaded for free from the PAHO website.

This guide notes that in the majority disasters, local groups are responsible for the management of human remains until specialist teams from outside, including forensic specialists, come in to help.

As I noted in the text, the Guide recommends that you appoint people specifically to the task of managing dead bodies. This might be possible only if you have a group of people organized as part of your sustainability efforts. In part this recommendation arises because some people simply will not have psychological reserve to deal with the stress of the situation. Others may not be able to handle physical demands of the work involved.

There are concerns about the spread of infection from dead bodies, and we know that most of this will be from contamination of drinking water supplies with fecal matter released from dead bodies. This is true in cases where a natural disaster such as earthquake or flood has caused death.

In the event of an infectious outbreak, it is possible for infection to occur if those who died were infected with a transmissible organism. Most infectious organisms, however, cannot survive on dead bodies after about two days, although the HIV virus can persist about six days afterwards.

Because of this, reasonable safety precautions to protect workers from blood and body fluids of the dead are mandatory. These include gloves and boots, aprons or gowns, and face masks. Handwashing, as well as disinfection of clothing, equipment and vehicles used to handle the dead bodies once the work is done are also essential.

Rapid recovery of bodies and placement in appropriate temporary storage is important, not just with regard to disease but also because it increases the likelihood that bodies will be identified correctly. It also helps in reducing psychological burden for survivors.

In circumstances when health care or other authorities are not available to help us, victims of a disaster need to be identified. To facilitate this process, the PAHO guide recommends labeling, photographing, recording and securing the bodies.

First, label each body on waterproof label (using a permanent marker) and securely attach it to the body inside the body bag or other wrap or container. You should also label the body container with the same number and record it in your documentation system.

Prior to storage , the body should be cleaned to allow identification of the face, but otherwise left in the condition in which you found it. Standing at the midpoint of the body, a photographer should take pictures including the whole face as well as a full-length view of the body from the front. Photograph any obvious distinguishing features, such as scars, deformities or tattoos. It's important to include the identification number in each of these photographs.

Once you have taken photographs, record the victim's gender, approximate age range, plus personal belongings found (including driver's license or other identity cards) and identifying features described above along with the number used to identify the body.

Finally personal items should be labeled and packaged and left with the body which should also be left in its clothing.

Ideally it is best to have two groups. One recovers the bodies and takes them to a centralized collection point, where they are identified as above. The second group could then take them to a storage site.

You should try to finish storage of human remains within 12-24 hours; otherwise decomposition will occur, which will impair later identification. Ideally, cold storage should be used, perhaps in refrigerated trucks or railcars. In other times, ice rinks have been used. You can also create a dry ice storage container by building a wall about 2 feet high around groups of 10-20 bodies and placing 20 pounds of dry ice (not in contact with any of the bodies) inside. This entire structure is then covered with a plastic sheet or tent. It is essential that you don't do this in an enclosed space, as the carbon dioxide given off by the evaporating dry ice could cause problems. A final option is to bury the bodies temporarily as described in the PAHO guidebook. Don't use ice as it could melt and create wastewater that may spread infection or hasten decomposition of the bodies.

Any event that causes widespread death and destruction will be stressful. Rapid, respectful handling of victims of these disasters will ensure the continued health of their loved ones and the community at large.

Injury Prevention

THE EPIDEMIOLOGIC TRANSITION HAS ALSO OCCURRED IN PART BECAUSE OF SYSTEMS: IF you get injured in an accident nowadays, you probably have access to an Emergency Medical Services system to take you to the hospital. You will be taken to a trauma center if your injuries are severe enough. Say what you will about the cost and other non-clinical aspects of the American health care system, the trauma care system is pretty impressive.

We know from Katrina and other major disasters, however, that depending on this system after disaster may be somewhat dicey. Even if things don't get really bad like that again, do you want to risk an injury changing your life forever despite the best care from our trauma system? We may find ourselves backpedaling, just as we may when it comes to infection. We have to focus on injury prevention, too.

Injury prevention isn't very sexy. Protection can go too far, I suppose: Nobody wants to be laughed at when they're out mowing the lawn in body armor, for example. We should really talk about risk reduction, not risk elimination. In this section, we will cover some very basic principles of injury risk reduction that apply to many of situations.

My first injury prevention principle is that you should leave your ego at the door. There are some things that you will be able to do, and others that you simply shouldn't try. I know of a doctor who takes care of a lot of older men who have been injured by falling off their roofs as they try to clean off leaves in the Fall. He reminds them "roofs are for roofers." Don't do things you aren't trained and equipped to do safely, under any circumstances!

When it comes to equipment, follow the safety instructions of the manufacturer. In our litigious society, product manufacturers are risk averse. This means that they will have thought of most of the things that could go wrong during the use of their products and have recommended measures you should take to prevent these mishaps. You should follow these instructions; if you think you look silly doing so, remember rule #1 about your ego. If that doesn't convince you, think how silly you might look *after* the mishap.

Consider, for example, that I have cut the clothes off of many motorcyclists in the ED after they come in from crashes. As I dig the sand and other grit out of their "road rash." not a pleasant experience for them, they tell me that long sleeves don't look cool.

Once, friends of a snowboarder told me he, like them, didn't wear a helmet because it didn't fit the "culture" and they couldn't get in boarding films. He couldn't tell me himself, because he needed me to intubate him (putting a tube in his throat and hooking him to a respirator) after he sustained a massive head injury.

Improvisation is a major sub-theme in this book. You may recognize that the piece of equipment or process you are using has a potential hazard or other shortcoming. If this is the case, and you are uncomfortable or queasy about how something might go, you may need to improvise a fix.

It snows a lot where I trained, and in the ED we had an informal "Day of the Snowblower" after the first big snowstorm. Typically on Day of the Snowblower, we had a rush of people, usually men, who mangled their hands trying to clean the chutes in their blowers that had been clogged by heavy wet snow. Many lost parts of fingers, or worse.

I know of one man who used a sturdy stick instead of his hand to clear blockages in his snowblower's chute, but not because he came to my ED with a mangled hand. I heard of him because he made the papers because after he died, he was buried with that stick!

I have taken care of a lot of people who have sustained injury after the unskilled use of "skill saws." Many would not have lost some of their parts if they had simply used a pusher stick to propel the piece of wood they were cutting and shaping through the path of the blade, rather than their hands.

So, improvisation is great, but be careful with it. Wisdom has it that the last words of a redneck are "Hey, y'all, watch this!!!" If it seems dangerous despite your improvisational ingenuity, and thus unwise, it probably is. Don't chance it unless lives depend on your success, and then make every effort to improvise safe processes.

Finally, how do you get to Carnegie Hall? Everyone who has ever taken music lessons knows the answer: Practice, Practice, Practice! What this means for injury prevention is this: "Dry lab" your task. Visualize how you will do the job. Be like the golfer or batter who takes a few practice swings. Do whatever practice you can in preparing prior to performing the task at hand. If it is a complex task, you may be able to identify safety problems and come up with preventive steps to apply in advance.

As an ER doctor, I may seem to be trying to put myself out of work, but believe me: I have plenty of customers. The cost to individuals, families and society from preventable injury is huge, and the impact on lives is truly tragic. Imagine how gridcrash might magnify such tragedy.

Disease Management

MAYBE YOU HAVE DIABETES, OR SOME OTHER CHRONIC DISEASE. NOW (BEFORE GRIDCRASH) IS the time to make sure you ready your health as much as possible. Don't take this too far. While some diabetics end up getting dialysis or kidney transplants in the long run, I am not advocating that you have these done "early" or pre-ventively. Instead, learn how to manage your disease.

What you do need to do is learn as much as possible about your disease and how to manage it "non-pharmacologically." Weight loss, exercise and dietary interventions may help reduce disease burden, and even your cost of medicines, before gridcrash occurs. Afterward, it may save your life.

The U.S. Department of Health and Human Services' Office of Disease Prevention and Health Promotion reports that nine out of ten adults in the U.S. lack the knowledge and skills needed to prevent disease and manage their own health. Try to be that "other" one adult, who does have the knowledge and skills, for the diseases that you or your loved ones have.

Disease management (DM) has been defined as "a system of coordinated health care interventions and communications for populations with conditions in which patient self-care efforts are significant."

Basically what this means is that doctors, employers, case managers and others have decided that YOU can have a major impact on the chronic illness(es) that you have. Much of this impact will come from so-called nonpharmacologic measures rather than medications; your main responsibility when it comes to medicines is to take them as prescribed.

Habits, as discussed in some detail in Chapter 2, are where you will be encouraged to make most of this impact. Other lifestyle issues, though, may play a role. The specifics of exactly which measures you need to apply in managing your disease obviously depend on which disease you have. Not all lifestyle efforts will have major impact on your disease, and not every disease will be amenable to these measures. Some will seem like "no-brainers" whereas others may not be well known, even to your health care provider.

The main impetus for DM among health care providers has been the hope of improving health, longevity and quality of life. The US government has also recognized the potential cost savings of DM, which has been demonstrated to be significant for a number of chronic illnesses. Because of this, don't be too surprised to see it coming your way, even if you don't choose to try it on your own. It just makes sense in an age of demographic imbalance caused by the baby boom, where a lot of older, sicker folks will need to get health care and there are fewer young, healthy workers are around to help fund it.

We have talked about the benefits of preparation for gridcrash, even if it doesn't occur. Learning about DM will allow the financial and health benefits of disease management to accrue to you, too. While both cost savings and better health are very laudable goals that probably make a lot of sense to you, too, there is another reason for talking about disease management in this book.

In the event of a bad gridcrash-like infrastructure disruption, you will reap the benefits of maximizing your health through DM prior to and after the event. You also can take some measure of control of your symptoms should more conventional care like medication become unavailable for a brief period or even a long time.

How can you do this? If you have a chronic disease, talk to your doctor, your local health department and your insurance company about DM for your condition.

Consider older DM techniques, too, long supplanted by miracles of modern medicine. The *Allen diet*, for instance, helped extend the life of some diabetics in the days before insulin.

You can also do internet searches with your disease name and the phrase "disease management." but be wary of internet information quality. A good starting place is the *Health Information Resource Database* sponsored by the Department of Health and Human Services of the US Government. Look for .edu, .org and .gov sites, as these *tend* to be the most reliable sources of information. See the end of the book for more ideas and resources.

You might also talk to your doctor to find out how the environment affects your illness, and how it might change after gridcrash.

Most physicians, given enough time, would be interested in your playing a more active role in understanding and managing your disease with them, even if it may seem a bit weird to them if they were to learn all the reasons you are doing it. Many large medical practice groups, hospitals and health insurers have health educators that could help you in these efforts, too.

Finally, there are textbooks on DM for health care providers and popular books for the rest of us that you may be able to find at your library or local used bookstore. Keep you brain active in looking around.

Health Management

NOT ONLY DO FOLKS WITH CHRONIC DISEASE HAVE TO WORRY ABOUT THESE ISSUES; IF YOU are healthy now, make efforts to stay that way. In most complex humanitarian disasters in the modern era, people die from infections. Pandemic flu and bioterrorism are just some of the other potential infectious nightmares we could face.

All of these potential threats make the issue of immunizations critical. Having shots up to date can protect you from a variety of infections. If you get a cut, having an up-to-date tetanus booster every few years can save you a trip to the doctor's office, urgent care or the ED.

Not enough people get flu shots, for a variety of reasons. I won't engage in the debate about vaccines except to say that I support them in all but a few circumstances. The benefits far exceed the risks. Let me tell you from painful personal experience that a no-foolin' case of flu is not any fun under normal circumstances.

There are other reasons that having flu vaccine might be useful, though. Let's say there is an outbreak of an infection one winter, like SARS or even anthrax, and you are sick. Doctors describe the symptoms of a wide array of diseases as "a flu-like illness." It might be easier for those treating you to identify your case as a result of the new infection, as opposed to the flu causing you similar symptoms, if you have gotten a flu shot.

You might also want to talk with your health department about other immunizations, typically given to travelers, which can protect you in the event of cholera outbreaks, etc. Measles and cholera kill lots of refugees and internally displaced populations around the world every year.

Don't forget your chompers in all of these preps. The U.S. Army learned during peacekeeping operations in the Balkans during the '90s what many travelers already know: Many dental issues lead to shorter trips, as troops had to be sent back to Germany in order to receive dental care because of complications from tooth decay, costing time and money. Remember Tom Hanks in *Castaway*? Get your teeth fixed now, and make plans for continued dental hygiene during bad times. You don't want to have to improvise unless absolutely necessary. See *Austere Dentistry* if you need more convincing!

Austere Dentistry TIP

PERHAPS THE FIRST ITEM IN A DISCUSSION OF IMPROVISED DENTAL CARE SHOULD BE prevention, just like we talked about planning and preparation before any discussion of providing medical care.

As we noted earlier, dental issues are major problems for travelers, and I can tell you as an "amateur dentist" that I see loads of people coming to the ED for pain and infection related to tooth troubles. They show up either because they have no insurance or no dentist is available. These folks all could have benefited from some of the preventive measures described below; if things get bad, we may also face similar struggles and need these tips. When the supply chain is broken and you have run out of your stock of toothpaste, what do you do? Baking soda can meet the abrasive function of the compounds in toothpaste. Vinegar mixed in cool pre-boiled water has been suggested as a good mouthwash. Dental floss can be used more sparingly, and you may also choose to try to re-use floss after cleaning it. A cloth held over a fingertip could suffice as a toothbrush. Indigenous peoples the world over have chewed on sticks and used the fibers generated in this fashion to clean their teeth, often using wood ashes for toothpaste.

Don't use your teeth as tools for anything but eating. Be careful with tough and hard foods, too; these are frequent offenders with broken teeth. If you insist on using your teeth as tools, bite with your eyeteeth or canines. These have the thickest covering of enamel which may offer some protection.

Given all of these options, you should be able to continue to practice reasonable levels of oral hygiene, and as we talked about last chapter, you hopefully have started to take care of any major dental problems now, so really bad things like abscesses and impacted wisdom teeth won't strike at an inopportune time. Despite all your efforts, though, a time may come when you have to take some of these matters into your own hands.

In the same way that you may choose to seek specialized training for yourself or someone in your community sustainability effort as a medical auxiliary, you may also choose to do this for dental care. This type of care may be all that you have available. Witness what happened in World War II: One man, who had dropped out of dental school and joined the army, became "dentist" for his POW camp after he was captured. He used his limited knowledge and the few tools at hand to perform over 10,000 tooth extractions!

Only one state in the US allows anyone other than a dentist to pull teeth or fill cavities. There are some proposals that would create the dental equivalent of nurse practitioners to provide care where dentists are in short supply.

Some dentists, though, have warned that even something seemingly simple like a tooth extraction could lead to serious complications. One dentist has testified that allowing dental auxiliaries these privileges "would be reproducing a level of patient care that America evolved away from years ago."

For a situation in which you find yourself unable to get dental care, like a long backpacking trip, or when our infrastructure is down, you should make plans to have some basic dental first aid supplies on hand; the list below is just one of many suggested lists out there. Some of these items will be duplicates with what you should have in a regular first aid kit.

With this kit, you will be able to treat pain, temporarily replace a filling or crown, stop most dental bleeding and possibly reimplant a tooth that had been knocked out, then stabilize it. You can download (free of charge) books like *Where There Is No Dentist* at a number of sites or Space Station protocols to keep with your emergency supplies as guidance.

■ Alcohol preps and Antibacterial towelettes
■ Pain medications: Acetaminophen, Ibuprofen
■ Tongue scraper
■ Oral antiseptic
■ Tea bags (moistened between gauze pads, then bitten to slow bleeding)
■ Anesthetic gel like Anbesol, Campho-Phenique or Orajel
■ Hydrogen peroxide (3%) or table salt (disinfectant gargle)
■ Temporary filling materials like Dent Temp or Tempenol

- Cotton swabs (Q-tips) and cotton balls
- Gauze pads (2 inch x 2 inch)
- Dental mirror
- Tweezers
- Oil of cloves (topical anesthetic)
- Stick of wax (to pad sharp teeth and stabilize loose teeth)
- Small plastic spatula
- Tooth picks (round)
- Instant ice pack
- Baking soda
- Aloe vera gel
- Wintergreen

Once you have made the decision to go further with acquisition of more skills and supplies, and you try to do things like tooth extractions and abscess drainage, you are crossing a Rubicon. Find ways to get as much training and experience as possible, perhaps helping at a free clinic or observing a veterinary dentist, then remember that these are techniques for true emergencies. Remember also that you could make things much worse if you don't do it right, and *nobody* will be around to bail you out. See the appendix for a suggested list of items for an advanced dental kit.

What can you do when trouble strikes you have dental issues and don't have formal supplies, and there is no dentist around? Here are a few suggestions.

Toothache: Any tooth pain indicates inflammation and possibly infection. In general, toothaches occur if tooth decay inflames or has penetrated into the pulp that contains the tooth's nerves. Toothaches can be caused by trapped food, so rinse the area with warm water to loosen whatever may be causing the pain.

Alternatively, a piece of cotton or gauze soaked in lime juice or oil of cloves can be placed on the tooth. Oil of cloves has some anti-bacterial properties, plus a remarkable numbing effect.

Over-the-counter pain relievers can help toothaches: ibuprofen, aspirin, acetaminophen and the like. Aspirin contains salicylic acid, which can burn and damage gums, so don't rub aspirin on your gums in hopes of numbing the pain. You could try pain-relieving gels like Anbesol or Orajel if available.

Other old home remedies for toothaches include: rinsing your mouth with salt water or dabbing some clove oil directly on the bad tooth. There may be a numbing power in cooled peppermint tea. Swish and swallow or spit.

Canker sores: Some toothpastes contain sodium lauryl sulfate, or SLS, that has been linked in some studies to the development of canker sores. Avoid eating sharp or jagged foods like chips, which can cause tiny cuts and scrapes in the gums and allow entry of a canker-causing virus.

Once you have a sore, garlic-laden foods seem anecdotally to help speed healing. Tea tree oil can be purchased in mouthwash form and applied directly to the site of the canker sore and may help to soothe inflammation.

Bleeding gums: A traditional home remedy is to bite down on a wet tea bag for bleeding gums, as well as tooth or gum pain. Teas contain tannins, which seem to shrink swollen tissue and help stop bleeding.

Tooth knocked out of its socket: It's said that for each minute a tooth is out of its socket it loses 1% of its chance of survival. Even teeth replaced rapidly may need root canals, so make sure you will have access to that level of service; if not, think twice about replacing teeth.

Shake or *gently* rinse off debris to avoid removing the important periodontal ligament, ideally by placing the tooth in a container of milk; try to reach a dentist within 30 minutes. If you can't, you need to numb the socket, remove the blood clot and re-insert the tooth. This takes some force, and a fractured tooth socket may cause problems. Once the tooth is back in place, you can use over-the-counter temporary dental cement (available in pharmacies) or warm wax (pre-mixed with a few fibers from a shirt to strengthen it) applied over the lost tooth and its neighbors to anchor it in position.

Broken tooth: If you see blood in the piece remaining in the mouth, the tooth has been broken into the pulp It will probably die and become an abscess; try to get to a dentist. Anbesol applied into the pulp may help deaden the pain.

If you can't, you can try to "caulk" the remaining tooth with softened sugar-free chewing gum if you don't have Cavit or a similar fix.

Sharpened teeth that haven't violated the pulp but have edges that can irritate or cut the tongue, lips or gums need to be filed down, with an emery board if available.

Something stuck between your teeth: Gentle brushing, flossing and rinsing may work to remove the object, but if it doesn't and the surrounding gum begins to swell, see your dentist if possible. The object may be bit of chipped enamel or a broken filling, and popcorn husks may occasionally need to be removed by a dentist.

Loss of a filling or crown: Cover with a temporary material and do not try to put the old filling back in the tooth. If you want to try to salvage a crown, you can try Vaseline, denture adhesive or over-the-counter temporary dental cement to hold the crown in place until you can reach a dentist.

Abscesses: Usually these must be drained, perhaps by inserting the point of a sterilized thin knife blade (ideally a sterile #11 scalpel). Snow or ice may be helpful to anesthetize the area. Pack the drained abscess cavity with clean gauze strips after you have rinsed it with salt water after all meals. Large abscess may lead to fever, and may lead to severe facial swelling that should be treated immediately to prevent airway compromise.

NOTE

We have talked a lot about habits in this book. Health effects aside, keep in mind that the day may come when your drug of choice, be it coffee, booze, smokes or pills, is no longer available. Some cynics even recommend stockpiling these items in advance of hard times to have something to barter. Seems like an ethical minefield to me, and although I recommend having some high-proof grain alcohol in storage, I don't foresee using it to tie one on. You'll have to keep reading to learn why.

Doing It on the Cheap

IN THESE HARD ECONOMIC TIMES, MANY PEOPLE WILL BE UNINSPIRED, UNWILLING OR UNABLE to undertake some of these measures due to cost issues. Some don't have health insurance. Some may not choose to prioritize purchases and keep supplies on hand. No one should be subjected to judgment or criticism for being forced down the path of poor preparedness by circumstance. Choices are also very individual, and if you choose not to heed any of the advice here, or to seek alternative options, that is your business.

If you are trying to do some of the prep work and planning described here, I hope that the lifestyle changes you institute do save you money and make you more healthy. Scavenging stuff legally, and reusing or repurposing other stuff, plus shopping for non-perishables during sales, using coupons, buying generic and making bulk purchases all may help cut costs.

Take advantage of inexpensive sources of care. Consider that many community colleges and technical schools have dental hygiene programs that are in need of patients for their students. Some offer cleanings for free. This kind of preventive care may also be available through other health schools: Many states have practical exams for dentists to get their licenses. I had friends who recruited patients for their dental school finals and actually PAID these patients to ensure they showed up on the appointed day. These and other opportunities may allow you to accomplish these preparedness activities at lower cost.

Conclusion:

Some old guy, Ben Franklin if you believe the historians, said that an ounce of prevention is worth a pound of cure, and in many cases, that ounce of prevention may indeed be worth a pound of flesh or more. Despite that, preventive efforts have lost a lot of their appeal in our modern, convenience-based society with its easy access to technological fixes. We are learning that some of those fixes may cause other problems. Even if they don't lead to problems now, there will be problems when those fixes are suddenly unavailable.

Don't wait until you really need them to learn about, practice and adapt the preventive measures we discussed in this chapter. They can save you time, gold or reputation now. Maybe they will save your life or the life of a loved one later, when the world as we know it has changed. In the next chapter, we will talk about how to reconstitute a health care system for you and those close to you when those big changes are happening all around us. ●

CHAPTER 5

Medicine When There Is No Doctor

Medicine When There Is No Doctor

IF YOU AREN'T NERVOUS, YOU AREN'T PAYING ATTENTION. I DON'T SEE MYSELF AS A PROPHET OF doom, but just the same I am nervous. As I write this, it seems that potential scenarios for hard times are in the news daily: the H1N1 outbreak and potential pandemic; one economic calamity after another causing Depression 2.0; Climate Change; Petrocollapse or Energy Descent; and plasma balls from the sun or other "space weather" events wrecking the electric grid via a Carrington Effect, just to name a few.

Any one of these happenings could disrupt the infrastructure of modern society. While some are preventable, with others we'll just be along for the ride. Prevention, though, would require buy-in from a lot of people in order for sufficient changes to occur to avert declines in our standard of living. I for one am not counting on those changes occurring.

Does that mean I am building a bomb shelter in my backyard, or storing coal in a pit somewhere, or hoarding gold? No. Nor does it mean I am totally blowing off efforts to have some planning and preparation in place for potential hard times.

On the other hand, if the Earth is like a vessel, we have to plan on having some form of lifeboat for troubled times.

The choice is yours: You can do as much or as little as you feel you need to. Maybe you have skills or stuff that you feel you can reasonably rely upon for barter. We have already witnessed the return of barter on a small scale in the US and the UK during the current recession. It is likely to return full-scale in the future. If you choose to rely on bartering for essentials like food, water, energy, or shelter, though, you must have a very desirable thing to offer in trade. Same goes for obtaining needed health care services. Alternatively, health care may be what you have to offer for barter for other goods and services at the flea market or town square.

Let's assume that you have already done the necessary preparation and planning. What other steps can you take now, and what can you do when the lights go out or the bottom falls out, to help reconstitute a medical care system, be it for your family or for your community? This chapter will focus on how to be self-reliant when the world as we know it is ending, or has come to an end.

Most self-sufficiency guides point to prior times: using old skills, materials and technology to live, things we have set aside as we have replaced self-reliance with the plethora of mechanization and technology. In seeking to meet your health care needs, you should focus not only on this adaptation of antique skills, but also on two more modern models: prisons and ships. Why these? Because they offer many useful handrails to guide our path to reconstituting an adequate health care system by ourselves.

I'm not talking about the modern, outsourced western prisons, but rather the open air prisons of the third world today, with latrines, wood fires for cooking and other more quaint features. We can learn a lot about meeting needs for food, water and shelter safely from the guidelines published for these prisons today.

Conversely, I am not talking about the old sailing vessels from the days of pirates and scurvy. Instead, I am talking about the modern oceangoing ships with a few crewmembers who have the additional duty of helping to provide some rudimentary care to crewmembers, and very advanced care in emergency, often with guidance from shore-based experts. Some of these "ships" will be spaceships, where crewmembers all have some training and are given protocols to follow along with guidance from earth-bound experts.

We will need all the guidance we can get if we are to find our way to a gentle landing as the world changes, or worse, falls apart. I hope the things we've discussed up to now will help you and that this chapter ties it all together for you. I will have advice on how you may go about stocking a facility for emergency health care, as might be planned by an intentional community, in advance of a time when there is no doctor. Finally, I will advise you a bit on improvisational medicine techniques you might be forced to use during the *really* hard times.

Prisons: Models for Sustainable Communities?

IN THE EVENT OF VERY BAD TIMES, WE MAY NEED TO REVERT TO TOTAL SELF-SUFFICIENCY: A small group or local community, we may need to be able to meet *all* of our needs for survival. Water, shelter, warmth, food, and health care (including sanitation) are the bare minimum. Do you know how much water you use daily? Do you know how to ensure it is safe to drink? For many of us, even if we knew this once upon a time, we may not know it now. It is simply a fairy tale to imagine we can conjure the knowledge and assume the burden when the time comes.

You can get a lot of this information for free by looking at guides published for other communities that have to be self-sustaining. One such guide is *Water, Sanitation, Hygiene and Habitat in Prisons* published by the International Committee of the Red Cross (ICRC). This guide describes how to meet basic human needs, and is available for free download at the ICRC website. It has pointers on minimum daily requirements and how to meet them with relatively simple (but labor intensive), and thus sustainable, techniques.

We know that health is more than just the absence of disease, and this guide will help you meet the bare necessities of life that are prerequisite to good health. Once you have a clean, warm place to live and everyone there has clean water and quality food, you will have gone most of the way towards good health. We have covered a lot of the needed measures, and this ICRC guide offers further knowledge to complement your emergency preparedness/ sustainability bookshelf.

Ships: A Guide for Your Medical Lifeboat?

MUCH OF THE KNOWLEDGE NEEDED BY A MEDICAL AUXILIARY IS OUT THERE, FREE OF CHARGE, for those willing to go out and get it. I am talking about books that are written for trained medical laymen who have "real jobs" that occupy their time but who also need to have some medical knowledge.

The International Maritime Organization, plus the US Coast Guard and similar agencies in other countries, require that ships with a certain size or crew complement have someone on board who can provide relatively advanced medical care whenever they set sail. As mentioned in Chapter 2, the Coast Guard has published *Standards of Training, Certification and Watchkeeping for Seafarers, to specify* the minimum standards needed for the "Medical Person-in-Charge" (MPIC) providing health care on ocean-going vessels.

If you are interested in sustainable health care activities for yourself, your family or your community, these standards are a great guidepost for the type and depth of medical knowledge you should seek to provide via your medical auxiliary. Most have been written by those who have provided care under austere circumstances. They have also been reviewed by medical authorities who are experts in the relevant subject matter.

Many guides also list supplies and equipment to help you choose what to have available for your medical auxiliary. Perhaps the biggest benefit of these books is their availability at low cost.

I hope that you have thought about taking the steps we talked about way back in the second chapter and have begun to prepare yourself, body, mind and spirit, for potential hard times ahead. As I've mentioned so many times before, and as our discussion of improvised medicine will reinforce, what you know means so much more than what you have. Still, it may pay to have some things on hand, just in case you need to reconstitute basic health care for those around you.

Medicines for Your Lifeboat

WHAT ABOUT HAVING OTHER MEDICATIONS LIKE ANTIBIOTICS, STRONGER PAINKILLERS AND the like on hand? You may choose, if you determine you have a potential need and are willing to invest the time, money and effort to be able to use them safely, to have a number of medications (usually obtained by prescription) on hand for a true gridcrash. Again, you must first know how to use this stockpile, which I call the *survival formulary*. See the appendix for a suggested survival formulary if you are designing an intentional community or other group to help if things get horribly bad. This list is designed to be efficient and modern, but will be limited to providing care for a small range of illnesses and injuries. It won't be a comprehensive list to allow you to care for chronic illnesses like diabetes and high blood pressure, for example.

The major obstacle in filling up your survival formulary is the issue of how you obtain the prescriptions needed to purchase most of these medications, to say nothing of the cost. Another issue, shelf life, is discussed in a previous tip.

Some "survivalists" and other preppers are well-known for recommending that you obtain prescription medications from animal supply stores, common to agricultural areas, or local pet stores so that you can provide advanced treatment of human beings without a prescription. These medicines include antibiotics like erythromycin, penicillin, tetracycline, sulfa and metronidazole that are used in fish tanks, for example, but are also used commonly to treat human beings. Although this is most assuredly a creative and brave strategy, I can't recommend it.

While it is certainly true that some medications used to treat animals are also used to treat humans, this is no guarantee that using medications produced for animals to treat people is in fact a safe practice.

The Food and Drug Administration monitors adverse drug reactions from veterinary medicines, including those that occur in human beings. Although production of animal medicine is regulated, there may not be the same level of purity in medications for animal use that is required for medicines destined for humans. Additionally, dosing can be drastically different and you could easily take too much or too little if you aren't cautious. Finally, there are also some situations in which human use of veterinary medications is actually illegal, although if things are too bad we probably won't have to worry about these legal niceties!

In terms of problems, there are medical literature reports that people who take animal medications have sustained bleeding ulcers, liver and kidney failure, anemia and other blood problems, seizures, respiratory failure and death. About 4000 people per year in the United States are poisoned by veterinary drugs. Some surveys showed that even veterinarians and other health care workers have taken medications designed for animals, although rodeo and horse racing participants seem to have a higher rate of this behavior. One report actually describes a dog owner taking medications intended for his dog in hopes of learning what kind of symptoms they were causing his pet. The same report also says, interestingly, that some of those taking animal medications were felt to be individuals with "more independent self-sufficient attitudes." Sounds like a group of people who might be reading this book!

One veterinary medication, phenylbutazone, or "bute," has been taken off the market for human use because of severe toxicity. Despite this, some folks continue to obtain it for use from animal supply stores, where it is sold in doses several times higher than typical human doses.

Based on all of this, I can't recommend that you take Fluffy's or Fido's medications. Even though some adventurous souls maintain that it is safe to do so, I think that at best this is hit-or-miss in terms of safety, and in some cases is downright foolish.

Another reputed source for drugs is by getting them from overseas, either from a neighboring country or via the Internet. The Food and Drug Act effectively prohibits legal importation of drugs into the United States other than by US-based manufacturers in most cases. Some personal importation is allowed but has to the based on the need for treatment of a serious condition, under the care of a physician, using medications not currently available at home. Even the re-importation of a drug produced in the United States and then shipped out of the United States is illegal, in fact a felony. Importation into the US of unapproved drugs that are used in other countries is a misdemeanor and could result in fines or imprisonment, even if the drug is approved for use in Canada or a European country.

If the foregoing legal proscriptions are not enough to convince you, keep in mind that the US Food and Drug Act is one of the strictest in the world and is designed to protect consumers from counterfeit, contaminated, outdated or low-quality medications. There are no such guarantees on medications made outside the US, as we have seen with the recent news about contaminated blood thinners and the deaths resulting from their use.

Another supposedly reliable source is obtaining medications during travel, most typically to Canada or Mexico (for people living within the United States). Keep in mind that there may be unscrupulous vendors willing to sell you substandard or out-of-date products in these circumstances.

One study in San Diego reported that people who got antibiotics over-the-counter in Mexico had high rates of drug reactions, whereas none of those who got them from Mexican pharmacies with a prescription had reactions. Some of these over-the-counter medications have made their way to the bodegas of New York City, where presumably they carry the same risk.

Regardless, in all of these circumstances, *caveat emptor* applies. Make sure that if you spend money you get what you pay for and that it safely meets your needs.

There has also been a recent explosion of online pharmacies where people can purchase their medications via the Internet. While this is useful for people who have access to a physician for prescriptions, as it may allow them to save money on medications, it is not without controversy.

Some Internet pharmacies have been known to sell controlled medications like narcotics to minors without safeguards, and there have been reports of people committing suicide with medications they obtained via the Internet.

Other services are famous for providing "lifestyle medications" such as erectile dysfunction drugs simply for a small fee after a potential recipient fills out an online form. There are other internet pharmacies providing other medications that would be much more useful to someone interested in providing ongoing medical care during hard times, though.

My recommendation is that if you choose to obtain medications for your survival formulary through an Internet pharmacy, it should be one based in your home country, ideally one in your home state. It should be one where the medication is provided after a physician reviews your request prior to filling the prescription; keep in mind that some of these online physicians review *hundreds* of these requests per day and they may miss important details about other medicines you are taking or your allergies.

Because of this, I strongly advise that you *do not* do this for routine medications that you or a loved one uses, and that you not use the medications obtained this way except under emergency circumstances. The usual checks and balances of having a physician prescribe medications, followed by a pharmacist's review of your other medications, allergies, drug interactions and other issues, have been removed.

Of all the options for obtaining medications for your survival formulary, I think getting them directly from your physician or other health care provider who knows you is best. Be honest about your reasons for doing this. Some folks say you could also tell your prescriber that you need them for travel or an expedition; just make sure they don't see you at the grocery store when you're supposed to be in Timbuktu!

Keep in mind that in most places dentists can prescribe the same medications as physicians; perhaps your dentist would be more approachable about this sort of project. Failing this, the Internet option is available but probably not the best.

I would strongly caution you against using overseas Internet pharmacies or trying to re-import medications from outside the country, in part because of potential legal ramifications, but primarily because of concerns about the safety and quality of the product you'll be taking.

Austere Hormones TIP

PRIOR TO THE 1920s, DIABETES KILLED MANY CHILDREN. ACCOUNTS OF THE ERA describe hospital wards full of comatose children gradually sliding into death, unable to fight off infection and dehydration, surrounded by grieving parents. Scientists and physicians had some understanding of what was going on in these children, but until 1922, were not able to do anything about it. Other diseases of *endocrine* (glandular) organs like the thyroid and adrenal glands, as well as sex hormones, have caused misery over the centuries, though not as much as diabetes.

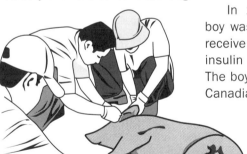

In 1922, one young teenage boy was chosen to be the first to receive an experimental injection of insulin purified from ox pancreas. The boy survived, and the group of Canadian researchers, led by Dr. George Blanding, won the Nobel Prize.

These early preparations of insulin were impure, resulting in allergic reactions and other complications. Later, pig pancreas was used to make insulin because it was less likely to elicit immune reactions in recipients. Finally, during the later decades of the 20th century, recombinant DNA "cloning" allowed production of human forms of insulin in vats of genetically engineered bacteria.

Obviously the latter is a high-tech, energy intensive and infrastructure-dependent product. If you know someone who is dependent on insulin, you should make sure they have extra on hand in the event of a short-term disaster that prevents them from getting new supplies; this applies to glucose testing and insulin administration supplies as well. Unfortunately, we don't have a way to provide another option like oral hypoglycemics for insulin-dependent diabetics to use right now.

But what happens in case there is a long emergency, where the supply chain is interrupted for a longer time, perhaps permanently? Do we have to revert to the bad old days of before Blanding and company?

In this setting, you may choose to try *oregano therapy*. This technique was pioneered by a French surgeon who used ground rooster testicle injections in hopes of restoring the lost vigor of his youth. He believed the testosterone contained in these injections would perk him up a little bit. Other clinicians extended these experiments and used animal organ extracts to treat diabetes as described above, as well as hypothyroidism that was so severe as to cause patients to lapse into coma and die.

If you have access to places where livestock are slaughtered for food, you could try to recreate the experience of these early researchers by making your own insulin and other hormonal substances like thyroid supplements. You may choose to read about how they made insulin from animal pancreas in the biomedical literature of the time. See the references for this chapter at the end of the book.

Similarly, those folks who take thyroid supplementation may have to go back to harvesting animal thyroid glands. They merely need to eat some of this organ, and also have the advantage of being able to take pills that probably have a longer shelf-life than insulin. Dosing of the glandular tissue would also be harder to figure out.

Adrenal hormones for folks with adrenal insufficiency may also be harder to make, but like thyroid medicines, they are available in a longer-lasting oral form. Similarly, birth control may be stored longer term. (See Tip on the SLEP to learn tips about how you might store and extend medicines beyond their expiration dates.)

For those who are worried about post-menopausal symptoms or prostate problems later in life, there is also hope. We know that a class of chemicals called *Phytoestrogens* found in soy products will reduce the incidence and severity of hot flashes and benign prostatic hypertrophy (enlargement), or BPH. Soybeans also have a good form of protein and can be used to make soy milk for baby formula, so you might want to be prepared to store and/or grow soybeans.

Any situation that forces us to return to using the Earth and its flora and fauna means that we may need to utilize all the resources available to us in order to sustain life and health. This includes using older formulations of hormones derived from animal products to treat many diseases, replacing the medicines we take for granted today.

Stuff: What to Have for When There Is No Doctor!

I THINK IT IS CLEAR TO YOU NOW THAT I DON'T RECOMMEND THAT YOU HAVE A BUNCH OF TOOLS that you don't know how to use safely and effectively. For one, having the tools without the knowledge may lull you into a false sense of complacency that you can use them as intended. Perhaps just as important, though, are the time, effort and money wasted in obtaining them.

For these reasons, I suggest that you have a good match between knowledge, skills and tools. Keep in mind that knowing when to do something is part and parcel of knowing how to do it and having the stuff to do it with!

Based on this practical philosophy, I have compiled a list of items that you might consider obtaining (see appendix), plus some suggestions on how to find them via non-traditional sources like eBay in the accompanying tip.

Village Hospital Items on eBay   TIP

LET'S SAY YOU'VE FOUND A GROUP THAT IS INTERESTED IN COMMUNITY SUSTAINABILITY, and you have decided that several of the members have or will acquire the training needed to act as medical auxiliaries in the event of a major emergency. How can you get the supplies needed to allow for more advanced care than simple first aid measures? Luckily, eBay comes to the rescue yet again.

On the same site where I found all those first aid supplies listed in an earlier Tip, I found the following more advanced supplies:

- Laryngoscopes
- Pulse oximeters
- Laryngeal mask airways
- Endotracheal tubes and tracheostomy tubes
- Ventilators and ventilator circuits
- Oxygen concentrators
- Intravenous catheters
- Glass (reusable) syringes
- Hemocytometers
- Microscopes
- Urinalysis dipsticks
- Gram stain kits
- Hemoccult slides
- Automated external defibrillators
- Electrocardiography machines
- Ultrasound machines
- Sterile gloves
- Basic surgical instruments and instrument trays
- Surgical skin staplers
- Dental instruments
- Penrose drains
- Surgical drapes
- Portable suction machines
- Surgical cautery machines
- Sterile disposable scalpels
- Dermabond skin adhesive
- Sutures
- Traction splints
- Bledsoe walking cast boots
- Crutches
- Gel splints and air casts
- Webrill and plaster casting rolls (often sold as a "hobby supply"!)
- Autoclaves

Prisoners of War: The Triumph of Improvised Medicine

PRISONERS, ESPECIALLY PRISONERS OF WAR, OFTEN FACE UNIQUE HEALTH CHALLENGES AND in response to these challenges have come up with some imaginative techniques that may be of use in hard times. They can also be a source of inspiration, as they demonstrate the creativity, courage and tenacity of those who put these techniques to use.

Medical officers in captivity have used a lot of the coping mechanisms we talked about earlier. They worked as a team in overcoming the obstacles they faced and refused to give up on doing their duties as physicians. Some operated on their captors when the care that the adversary was able to provide was sub-par.

They observed the many manifestations of vitamin-deficiency diseases and conducted experiments that compared the relative efficacy of rice polishings, yeast or grass soup in patients with mouth ulcers due to riboflavin deficiency. They found that grass soup was the best treatment. Even in the midst of their captivity, they contributed to the advancement of their profession's knowledge, and their informal research setting did not prevent them from later publishing knowledge gained about the importance of riboflavin in preventing amblyopia, the loss of the center of one's visual field.

In the Warsaw Ghetto created by the Nazis to house Polish Jews prior to sending them to the concentration camps, a number of physicians took this desire to continue some semblance of normalcy to the utmost: They ran an underground medical school. Even though the eventual plan of the Nazis came to fruition, some of the students survived to practice medicine and other health specialties after the war. Others taught hygiene to the local populace in hopes of preventing disease that made the misery worse.

Frequently we have reports of prisoners using humor as a coping mechanism. Leo Thorsness, who was a POW in the Vietnam conflict and later a congressman, describes how his camp held a contest to see who had the most boils on their skin. Other camps used mosquito netting and other rags to make theatrical costumes for plays that boosted morale.

In many prisons, the basic diet provided to prisoners was deficient in calories, protein and vitamins, and resulted in rapid weight loss. Many prisoners also developed a whole range of problems due to vitamin deficiencies: edema of the legs and heart failure, painful fissures of the mouth and scrotum, rashes, painful burning feet, inflammation of nerves and poor vision.

Their situation required that prisoners be ingenious about securing every last milligram of vitamins in their rations, and also finding nutrients from other sources. Rice polishings, soy beans, (which were soaked in water and ground down to provide soy milk) pine needles, grass and green leaves (crushed into a pulp that was extracted with cold water) and other measures helped prevent thousands of deaths among prisoners whose daily diet often amounted to only around 500 calories.

Circumstances also forced prisoners, especially led by the doctors and dentists, and other imaginative types among them, to improvise tools out of what little their captors provided.

Under prison camp conditions, good hygiene was life-saving. Many camps made stills out of bamboo and put them to use to purify drinking water. Other camps also distilled alcohol in order to clean the hands of the surgeon as well as the skin of the patient prior to operation. There are many examples of very imaginative redirecting of materials toward medical use: Metal ration cans and other scraps were used to make burners for sterilizing instruments; prisoners made soap using wood ash and available vegetable oils or animal fats; and surgical tools were fashioned from tableware.

Surgical instruments were typically very hard to come by, so metal dinner knives were ground and sharpened into scalpels, forks were used as retractors and spoons were sharpened for use in curettage, or scraping out, dead and infected tissues; these spoons were credited by camp doctors with allowing them to forego some limb amputations. Even in the 1990s, surgeons in the Balkan civil wars continued this practice and used kitchen utensils as makeshift surgical instruments!

Dysentery and cholera were serious problems for prisoners in the camps of Southeast Asia during World War II, causing severe dehydration in some patients. Charcoal, chalk and bark teas were all used to reduce diarrhea from cholera and dysentery and to treat intestinal parasite infestations.

Prisoners made saline solution from rainwater, or with river water that they had filtered. In the larger camps, improvised stills were used to purify water for intravenous use. IV bottles were made from empty wine or beer bottles whose bottom ends the detainees cut off. The neck was capped with a wooden cork and a hole was made in the stopper. Then, a piece of bamboo was inserted into the hole and the outlet was connected to stethoscope tubing. The IV needle, or cannula, was often carved from a piece of a hollow bamboo spine. In some cases, saline was also given through the rectum.

Blood transfusions were often lifesaving. A Canadian surgeon developed a simple technique of stirring blood with a bamboo stick or whisk for 10 minutes. This caused the fibrin in the blood, which ordinarily would have forced it to clot in a gelatinous mass, to collect on the stick itself. The defibrinated blood was then filtered through layers of gauze and administered through the type of IV set described above.

One Dutch doctor made a microscope using bamboo and binocular lenses that was good enough to enable blood typing as well as the diagnosis of some large parasites like the cause of malaria.

Bamboo trunks were split, then strapped around broken limbs in lieu of plaster casts. Clean nails or sharpened bicycle spokes were inserted through bones as traction pins, and bags of sand used as weights for placing fractures in traction to allow correct healing.

In another very memorable instance, reported by an Australian POW surgeon, homemade sake (the distilled alcoholic beverage) allowed production of a general anesthetic. He needed to operate to ligate an aneurysm on one of his fellow POWs, working deep under his patient's shoulder to do so. Unfortunately, his captors refused to provide him with any anesthetic.

He turned to another prisoner, a Dutch pharmacist, (or chemist as they were then known) and asked for help. The chemist requested two basic materials: ethyl alcohol and sulfuric acid. He was given alcohol from some bootleg rice sake that a few enterprising prisoners were making in their hut, and battery acid, stolen from the auto shop where some prisoners worked, supplied the other component. Two weeks later, the product, ether, was available and the operation went forward. In all, they made enough ether to perform over 40 more surgeries!

Dental care under these circumstances also often left something to be desired. Thorsness and his fellow prisoners often chipped teeth or lost fillings on the rough foods they ate in captivity. Sometimes they got bread instead of rice; once he noticed a piece of bread had gotten stuck in one of his cavities, and that the pain from the cavity was dulled with the bread in place, so he left it there. Word got around, and he and several others often used bread for temporary fillings!

While your "when there is no doctor" style improvised medicine might not be practiced under conditions this harsh, the hardiness, ingenuity and skill of these medical POWs provide us with a great model showing how we can use older techniques and simple materials to provide good health care in hard times or bad places.

Medicines from Nature: The Original Sustainable Medicine

IN THE LAST FEW DECADES, MANY FOLKS HAVE TURNED TO A NUMBER OF COMPLEMENTARY and alternative medicine (CAM) techniques like bodywork, meditation and herbal remedies out of frustration with modern medicine: Its cost, impersonal doctors or other frustrations are often at the root of this movement away from strict acceptance of doctor's orders. Others may doubt the safety and effectiveness of synthetic drugs. As of the year 2000 or so, 40% of Americans used some form of CAM; worldwide, that figure is closer to 80%. Even the National Institutes of Health, which were largely responsible for driving the development of scientific medicine in America, now has its own center for the study of CAM.

I am not unique among physicians when I say that I believe herbal medicine has many roles now. *Integrative medicine*, as pioneered by Dr. Andrew Weil, is the combination of allopathic (traditional) medicine with CAM. I am also not that unusual in that, while I understand that medicinal herbs have roles for many people and that many patients use them, I am concerned about a certain "snake oil salesman" element I see in a lot of the promotional efforts for these products. Finally, while I tend to be somewhat skeptical of some of the claims made with regard to the power of herbs, I hope that efforts to prove the efficacy of these medicines continue.

Believe it or not, most doctors don't sit around with each other, or with reps from the drug companies, discussing how to stifle attempts to bring useful medicinal plants to people's attention. On the contrary: If we can be convinced that the benefits of these natural products outweigh their risks and other disadvantages, we would certainly use them. Remember that a lot of what we use now came from nature: aspirin, penicillin and digitalis, just to name a few.

The reality though, is, that medical practitioners are under increasing pressure to use good quality published evidence in making decisions about diagnosis and treatment. As the former editor of the *Journal of the American Medical Association*, George Lundberg, once said, there is no alternative medicine, just *good* medicine based on evidence. Unfortunately, except in rare instances, there just isn't a lot of published evidence, pro or con, when it comes to herbs.

Having said all that, I also recognize that during hard times or after a crash scenario, many of our conventional medications may not be available. During these times, it will be essential to have other mechanisms in place to provide medications to those who need them. Stockpiling drugs in advance is all well and good, but may not always be feasible due to the amount and wide range of medications that could be needed, not to mention the cost and other logistical issues.

For all of these reasons, a discussion of basic herbal medicine is essential. If this is an area of interest for you, I have enclosed a list of resources in the appendix for this chapter that you can use to educate yourself. I also suggest that you speak with knowledgeable herbalists to learn about wild herbs that can be found in your area, as well as to learn what kinds of medicinal plants can be cultivated where you live.

Skill and facility with herbs as well as knowledge of their application and effects have traditionally been in the realm of spiritual healers and barefoot doctors, as well as traditional healers in the recent past. In addition, in Europe, Asia and other parts of the world, herbal medicine continues to have widespread application, out of tradition or necessity, and has a growing body of research to support it.

Knowledge of herbal medicine falls into two areas that could be mutually exclusive, or one person could try to become expert in both: botanical knowledge and therapeutic knowledge. As with a lot of information needed for sustainable living, both were common knowledge in the past. Anthropologists point to a large body of evidence suggesting herbal medicine was well developed in ancient societies.

Botanical knowledge includes recognizing and cultivating medicinal plants, while therapeutic knowledge comprises knowing what herb does what and how to compound the product to get the active ingredient where it needs to go. You can learn more about how to make your herbs into medicines from *Making Herbs into Medicines*.

HERBAL REMEDIES CAN OFTEN BE MADE FROM HERBS THAT ARE EASILY FOUND AT ANY grocery store, food co-op or natural food store. Pharmacies might have some herbal items as well. Finally, you might find living plants like Aloe Vera at gardening stores, greenhouses, or growing outdoors on a farm or in the wild.

Once you have your herbs, you will need a dosage form in which the active ingredient will be easily, and hopefully palatably, available to your patient's system. Some of the ways you can prepare herbs include:

Infusions: These are your typical teas. You can even use a metal tea strainer to help you make them. Add 1-2 teaspoons of dried herb (2-4 teaspoons of fresh) to a cup of boiling water. Infuse for 10 minutes before discarding the herb, straining the infusion if need be. Some infusions will become bitter if allowed to steep too long. Don't make these sooner than one day in advance as they can lose potency.

Decoctions: Are for more resistant materials like bark and seeds. Add 1-2 teaspoons to a cup of cold water and bring to boil. Cover and simmer for 10 minutes.

Tincture: Put 4oz of a dried herb into a glass jar, add 2 cups clear alcohol like grain alcohol or vodka and cover with lid. Let this sit in the dark for 2 weeks, shaking occasionally, then strain through a cheesecloth into a brown glass bottle to limit light exposure. (*This* is the reason you should have some high-proof alcohol like grain alcohol in your survival supplies, not for partying. If you want that, there are loads of guides on how to homebrew wine, beer, mead, and other alcoholic drinks for yourself.)

Syrup: Start with 2 cups of strained infusion, decoction, or tincture of an herb. Add 1¾ cup brown sugar or honey. Heat until sugar dissolves or honey is thin. Place in a bottle, seal, and refrigerate. Honey helps act as a preservative, and both honey and sugar offer some flavoring.

Steam: Add a strong decoction or 2 teaspoons of a tincture to boiling water. Pour into a pot, then cover head and pot with towel. Inhale steam.

Oil Infusions: Fill a jar with a fresh herb then cover with olive oil. Place the jar into a pot of warm water with the waterline above the level of the oil. Simmer for about 3 hours and strain through filter paper or cheesecloth into a brown glass bottle. Cool prior to use. For EXTERNAL USE ONLY.

Ointment or Salve: Melt 4 parts plain Vaseline-type petroleum jelly or olive oil using a double boiler and add 1 part herbs. Melted jelly should cover herbs completely. Stir mixture. Strain into jars while hot. Ointment is ready to use when cool. For EXTERNAL USE ONLY.

Compress or Poultice: Soak a washcloth in a warmed infusion or decoction of herb, wring out the cloth carefully and apply to affected area. You may repeat when the cloth is cool. For EXTERNAL USE ONLY.

Plaster: These are good for skin infections and sprains. Mix ground herb or seeds with a small amount of boiling water to make a pulp. Place pulp in cloth and apply to affected area while warm. Replace when cool. For EXTERNAL USE ONLY.

A doctor of naturopathy (ND) would be a key person to aid you in learning the practice of herbal medicine, as that is a major component of what NDs do. If you are motivated by herbal medicine, then naturopathy school may be the place for you to get much of this know-how, and would also be a potential career avenue should you choose to follow it. Many schools of naturopathy have correspondence courses; some naturopathy programs also offer training as a naturopathic physician assistant.

You can also find naturopathy lectures on sites like YouTube and iTunesU; there are also recurring podcasts on natural medicine on iTunes.

If you choose to include herbal medicine in your plans for providing health care to yourself and loved ones in the event of hard times, keep in mind that this is an area that, like traditional medicine, requires that you obtain proficiency with a large body of knowledge in order to be safe and efficacious. Some of this knowledge mirrors that which Western medicine utilizes, like anatomy, physiology and infectious disease.

Keep in mind that some foods have tremendous value as medicines, as described in the nearby tip.

Remember, too, that many of the herbs used today in treatment are proven to be effective, while others are not. You might look into getting a copy of the *Commission E Monographs* on herbal medicine from Germany, where a lot of people use herbs routinely for maintaining health and treating illness. Finally, make sure that you can grow or obtain locally those herbs you intend to use in the event that shipping is impacted.

Improvised Medicine: When Nothing Else Is Available

WHEN YOU TREAT ANY ILLNESS OR INJURY, YOU TYPICALLY TREAT THE SYMPTOMS AS WELL AS the cause. In many cases, supportive care is all you need to carry a patient through the illness, allowing the body to recover on its own. This is true for many viral illnesses, a number of injuries, and even for some bacterial infections in very healthy individuals.

There is some debate among the proponents of "evolutionary medicine" about the appropriateness of simply treating symptoms rather than allowing them to occur. This argument stems from the concept that many of the body's reactions are in fact solutions or evolutionary coping mechanisms designed by nature to allow the body to fight off disease and heal itself.

Exemplifying this, fever is felt to help limit the growth of infectious organisms due to the higher body temperature, which helps the body's own chemical reactions to occur more quickly and efficiently. On the other hand, it can lead to seizures among other complications, beyond just making you feel miserable. Likewise, vomiting and diarrhea limit the ability of a toxin or infection to dwell in the gut and be absorbed to cause more problems, while leading to dehydration and other problems.

There is no conclusive evidence that treating symptoms harms a person's ability to fight off disease; some argue that at least with symptomatic treatment that people will be functional and feel better. In light of that kind of approach, you may need some simple, austere, or improvised means of treating common symptoms. In some cases, these treatments may also fix the underlying cause; keep in mind that you need to make sure that the patient is actually getting better, not simply feeling better because their symptoms are being masked.

In other circumstances, you may have no choice but to treat the injury or illness, as the complications from an infected wound, for example, are too dangerous to allow to occur unfettered.

The following list of improvised treatments is by no means comprehensive. Older folks can be valuable sources of knowledge, as can books like the Foxfire series and articles published in outdoor and self-sufficiency magazines.

These ideas are for times when you don't foresee having *any* access to modern supplies during the time period they are needed for your patient. Remember: These tips are for *no-fooling emergencies under very austere circumstances*. Always use materials prepared non-commercially with caution!!!

Fevers. You could treat fevers with tea made from willow bark, an infusion of elder flowers or fruit, linden flower tea, or elm bark decoction. These will contain variants of acetylsalicylic acid, or aspirin. Because of this, these treatments are not suitable for children due to the association of aspirin with Reye Syndrome.

For children whose temperatures exceed 102-103°, you can use tepid sponge baths with water. Do NOT use rubbing or other alcohols. The trick is to provide cooling without inducing shivering, which could cause more heat generation and worsen the fever, plus make your patient feel worse.

Nausea and vomiting. Ginger has been used for thousands of years in cooking, plus medicinally in folk and home remedies. Ginger, given as a capsule containing 250mg of powdered ginger root up to four times per day, is known to reduce nausea resulting from pregnancy and after surgery. It has not been proven, yet, to help if these symptoms are due to other causes, but if it's all you got, it probably won't hurt either.

Diarrhea. This common, debilitating symptom can be caused by a change of diet, drinking contaminated water, eating spoiled food, or using dirty dishes. Most of these causes can be avoided by practicing good hygiene. Peppermint tea has recently been shown to reduce the severity and frequency of symptoms attributed to irritable bowel disease. Another tea that offers beneficial effects on the gut is chamomile: A teaspoon of this common soother can relax the spasms of babies' intestines to lessen colic. It may also ameliorate the cramps in cases of diarrhea.

Diarrhea from colitis like Crohn's disease may be hard to care for without medicines. Green tea contains substances (catechins) that have been shown to reduce inflammation in animal models of inflammatory bowel diseases like Crohn's disease and ulcerative colitis.

If you develop diarrhea despite these measures, and do not have any anti-diarrhea medicine, one of the following treatments could be effective:

■ Limit your intake of foods for 24 hours. Sip clear liquids in small volumes frequently to avoid dehydration. After that, follow a low-residue diet: BRAT or bananas, rice, applesauce and toast is one such approach.

■ Teas made from the roots of blackberries and their relatives, and from cowberry, cranberry or hazel leaves may also work, too.

■ Drink a mixture of a handful of ground chalk, white clay, powdered wood charcoal or ashes (not from treated lumber or commercial briquettes), or powdered bones (best if burned and ground) with a cup of clean, treated water. If you have some apple pomace (the solid remains of fruits after they are pressed for juice or oil, containing the skins, pulp, seeds, and stems) or the shredded rinds of citrus fruit, add an equal portion to the mixture to increase its effectiveness. Use 2 tablespoons of this solution every 2 hours until the diarrhea slows or stops. Yummy!

■ When nothing else is available, drink one cup of strong tea every 2 hours until the diarrhea slows or stops. Tannic acid in teas can help to limit diarrhea. You can make these teas by boiling the inner bark of a hardwood tree like White Oak for at least 2 hours in order to release the tannic acid. You must use caution with this method as tannic acid can cause inflammation of the liver!

Intestinal Parasites. These nasties may be diagnosed by seeing something waving at you, so to speak, from your stools. You might also notice itching in a socially awkward location. Finally, a heavy burden of intestinal worms may lead to malnutrition, malaise and anemia.

You can avoid picking up worm infestations and other intestinal parasites if you practice prevention. The easiest way to prevent these parasites is to avoid under-cooked meat and raw vegetables contaminated by raw sewage or human waste used as a fertilizer. Never go barefoot. If you should become infested and lack proper medicine, you can try these remedies. Keep in mind these home remedies are intended to change the worm's environment within the gastrointestinal tract.

■ Salt water. Dissolve 4 tablespoons of salt in 1 liter of water and drink. Try this only once (as if you'd want to do it more than that!).

■ Tobacco. Eat 1 to 1 ½ cigarettes. Their nicotine will kill the worms or stun them long enough that your system might be able to pass them. If the infestation is severe, you could repeat the treatment, *but not before 24 to 48 hours after the first try.*

■ Kerosene. Drink 1 to 2 tablespoons of kerosene. If necessary, you can repeat this treatment in 1 to 2 days. Do not inhale the fumes as they may cause lung irritation.

■ Hot peppers. Hot peppers create an environment that is prohibitive to parasitic attachment and may be effective, but only if they are a steady part of your diet. Eat them raw or in prepared dishes.

Constipation. You may be able to relieve constipation by drinking decoctions made from dandelion leaves, rose hips, or walnut bark. Eating raw daylily flowers might also help. It's best to try to prevent this malady by staying hydrated, being active (walking, if you can't do anything else) and consuming fiber from fresh fruits and vegetables.

Bladder infections. Bladder infections will cause painful urination or burning with urination, a sense of incomplete emptying of the bladder and need to urinate more frequently than normal. You may also notice cloudy or bloody urine. Beyond these symptoms, kidney infections may cause flank pain, fevers and chills, and nausea and vomiting.

There is evidence that cranberry juice, and perhaps blueberry juice, will help prevent and treat bladder infections. These juices prevent certain types of bacteria from attaching to the wall of the bladder and may lessen your chance of infection. One study had patients suffering from bladder infections drink cranberry juice, and showed that about half improved significantly, while one fourth had no change.

Pneumonia/bronchitis/cough. Suspect pneumonia or bronchitis when a person has at least two of these symptoms:

■ A new cough, or a cough that changes character
■ Sputum production, or change in its amount or color if cough is chronic
■ Fever or shaking chills
■ Chest pain that worsens with breathing
■ Shortness of breath

If you have a pulse oximeter in your supplies, you may also detect low oxygen saturations in a patient with significant pneumonia.

The mainstay of therapy for bronchitis and pneumonia will be plenty of bed rest and fluids, therapeutic coughing and deep breathing exercises (to open the lungs and mobilize the infected material), proper diet, cough suppressants to allow rest (see *Honey As Medicine*), pain relievers and fever reducers, like aspirin (not for children) or acetaminophen; see above for austere fever remedies.

Humidity helps with some conditions, especially croup, the seal-like bark of its victims being a giveaway to the diagnosis.

If a person is severely ill from pneumonia, they may benefit from IV hydration, or proctoclysis if needed. (Described in *Fluid Administration without an IV*) Finally, if you have oxygen or an oxygen concentrator, this may be of benefit.

TIP | **Fluid Administration without an IV**

FLUID LOSSES OCCUR WITH A NUMBER OF DISEASE PROCESSES, INCLUDING FEVER, vomiting, diarrhea, bleeding or burns. If fluid losses are severe enough, death or severe organ damage can result if the fluid is not replaced rapidly. Even in cases of minor fluid loss, secondary symptoms like nausea, headaches, weakness, dizziness and fatigue can result, making your patient miserable.

As we talked about in an earlier chapter, intravenous access ("starting an IV") is something that could be learned and practiced using the gelatin intravenous model, but some folks may not be willing to acquire this knowledge, then practice and retain the skills required. Any dehydrated patient, especially children and the elderly, can present a challenge to the most experienced IV starter. Additionally, sterile IV needles, tubing and solution are not always going to be available under austere circumstances.

In some cases, in the absence of intravenous fluid technique and supplies, patients can be given oral rehydration adequate to meet their needs for fluid replacement. In the event a person is conscious and not vomiting, oral rehydration using salt solutions (developed by the World Health Organization for treatment of cholera victims; see /figure) make an excellent, easily made solution that will replace fluid and salts lost from diarrhea, severe burns and febrile illnesses like pneumonia and influenza. Pedialyte is one commercially available fluid that could be put to this use as well.

Once you have made your rehydration solution, give it slowly, for instance with a teaspoon. The goal is frequent, but small, sips. You may need to do this every 3-5 minutes. Adults may be able to drink 2 ounces every 15 minutes.

If your patient vomits, wait 10-15 minutes and give another few sips. Despite vomiting, some of the fluids and salts will be retained.

Extra fluid should be given until the vomiting and diarrhea have stopped, and urine is light rather than dark. This will usually take between three and five days.

Sometimes, though, patients will be unconscious or have injuries that will prevent them from absorbing fluid from the stomach, or they simply may be too nauseous to keep fluids down. Under these circumstances, an alternative to the oral route for hydration must be available if fluids cannot be given intravenously.

Prior to the advent of intravenous fluid administration, physicians and surgeons utilized a rather funny sounding technique for rehydration: proctoclysis. This austere fluid administration tool is useful in cases where your patient is unconscious or vomiting, and involves infusing fluids via the rectal route. This technique has been used by servicemen in previous wars, by mountaineers in the remote Himalayas, surgeons in Africa and by hospice for cancer patients who are dehydrated and unconscious or otherwise don't want to go through the discomfort of intravenous fluid administration.

The technique is simple enough: A flexible, soft and thin plastic tube such as a Foley catheter or nasogastric tube is gently inserted (after lubrication) about 1-2 feet into the patient's rectum and tap water or a salt solution such as Gatorade or Pedialyte is infused by gravity (the container held above the level of the patient) via the catheter into the patient's colon. Obviously, if the patient has diarrhea or bloody stools this technique should be avoided.

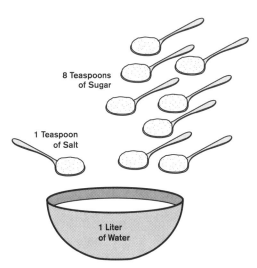

8 Teaspoons
of Sugar

1 Teaspoon
of Salt

1 Liter
of Water

One of the major functions of the colon is reabsorption of fluids secreted by the stomach and small intestine in the process of digesting food, so it's only natural that the colon would be excellent for absorption of other fluids, and in fact it's been shown that even in children the colon can absorb anywhere from 100-400 milliliters (5-13 ounces) of fluid per hour, which is a reasonable rate in all but the most extremely dehydrated patients.

By contrast, the average enema is about 6 ounces given over only a few seconds. The slow rate of instillation of the fluid in proctoclysis allows absorption to occur; the enema effect is observed in only few patients who undergo proctoclysis. In addition, the colon is able to assist the kidneys in correcting salt imbalances by selective absorption of the salts contained in the fluids.

Obviously the preferred route for any urgent fluid resuscitation is by IV infusion. As noted above, this requires sterile saline and other supplies as well as fairly sophisticated and somewhat perishable skills that may not be available to everyone. Because of this, using the natural route for absorption of fluids through the gastrointestinal system, whether delivered the usual way through the mouth and stomach or the antiquated technique of proctoclysis via the large intestine, is a viable alternative to the medically and technically intensive technique of the IV

*Some recipes recommend ½ teaspoon of baking soda, but this is not essential. It may help patients with profound diarrhea.

Sore throat/URI. Fever reducers will also help these symptoms, as will rest and extra fluid intake. Gargling warm water with salt, 1 teaspoon per pint, every few hours will help. Vitamin C is commonly recommended, and may help.

Burns. See the previous Tip detailing the use of honey in burn care. Aloe Vera is another widely available treatment, a plant whose sap helps alleviate the pain of burns, including sunburn.

Tannic acid from teas (allowed to cool, obviously!) made from tree bark seems to help limit the risk for infection in burns. The following burn treatment relieves the pain, seems to speed healing, and offers some protection against infection:

■ Soak dressings or clean rags for 10 minutes in a boiling tannic acid solution (made from tea, or the inner bark of hardwood trees or acorns boiled in water).

■ Cool the dressings or rags and apply them to burned areas.
■ Treat for shock by replacing lost fluid. For large burns, this could be a huge amount; the patient usually will report thirst. They should be urinating normal amounts and if not, may need more fluids.

Lacerations: Open wounds are dangerous in any situation, in part because of blood loss and tissue damage, but also if they become infected. Bacteria on the object that caused the wound, on skin and clothing, or on any foreign material and dirt that contacts the wound may cause infection, including tetanus in those without adequate protection from immunization.

You can reduce further contamination and promote healing by taking proper care of open wounds as soon as possible after they occur by:

■ Removing clothing (cutting it away as needed) from the wound.
■ Looking for exit wounds if a sharp object or bullet or other projectile caused the wound.
■ Cleaning the skin around the wound thoroughly with soap.
■ Irrigating the wound with large amounts (at least 4 ounces per inch of length) of water under pressure. See *Expedient Wound Irrigation* for more information on fluids to use. Use fresh urine if water is not available; urine will essentially be sterile if a person doesn't seem to be having symptoms of a kidney or bladder infection.

Expedient Wound Irrigation   TIP

DISASTERS WILL RESULT IN WOUNDS, INCLUDING SCRAPES, CUTS AND BURNS. THIS IS true whether the disaster actually causes the injury itself, or if recovery or long-term sustainability efforts after the disaster result in injury despite the best injury prevention efforts as described in the text. The next bad event that can befall the proud new owner of these wounds is infection.

In light of this, we need to consider infection control efforts that we can utilize after injury. For wound care, as we discussed in the ventilation section of the Chapter 4, dilution will be part of the solution to pollution.

Irrigation of wounds is a key step to the prevention of infection, which in turn will maximize the chances of a wound healing without too much pain, or functional or cosmetic impact.

How do you do irrigate wounds? Consider that in most hospitals, sterile fluids such as saline irrigation are used. These are expensive, sometimes hard to obtain, and will probably be in short supply for most people following a disaster. Luckily, there are alternatives.

One method is to use water treated with bleach. Clean tap water or bottled water can be treated with household bleach, resulting in wound irrigation that is sterile and non-toxic, and that may actually have bacteria killing effects left over from the bleach.

What's more, in 2004, military surgeons obtained water from lakes, ponds and creeks. They treated the water with 1 teaspoon (or 5 mL) of common household bleach per Liter of water. After this treatment, it appears the only one out of 100 samples contained any bacteria, and this was felt to be a contaminant from the air picked up during testing. Based on this, they offered their technique as a field expedient method for obtaining water suitable for irrigation of wounds.

Extending upon this work, an orthopedic surgeon at the University of Missouri showed that patients with open (or compound) fractures of the legs had no difference in outcome, and in fact had fewer wound healing problems, if they were treated with an irrigation solution made from nonsterile tap water and Castile soap rather than water containing the antibiotic bacitracin.

Alternatively, you can purchase distilled water and store it at room temperature. If you need it for irrigation, add a tablespoon of table salt to each gallon and use this as your irrigation fluid. Even when made by non-health care providers, if stored in the refrigerator at or below 48°, these solutions remained sterile for three weeks. This essentially reproduces the expensive sterile saline you can buy from your pharmacy.

Finally, a group from the State University of New York at Buffalo showed that water straight from the tap was just as effective at preventing wound infections as sterile saline when used for irrigation of wounds. Obviously, if this were adopted by other health care institutions, the potential savings would be huge. Unfortunately, medicine is often described as a profession where 200 years of tradition are untrammeled by progress. Additionally, patients often value the "totems of medicine." like use of sterile fluid.

Regardless, things happen, so keep in mind that if you're in a pinch, making your own irrigation fluid with a pinch of salt or a few drops of bleach works just as well and offer a lot of advantages over commercially made irrigation solutions in the fight against infected wounds.

You can use a clean plastic bag or plastic bottle; fill the container with the fluid, then close the container. Next, puncture it once or twice with a needle, then squeeze the container to create a "water pik" type jet and move the stream back and forth over the wound, rinsing out dirt and potential infection.

The "open treatment" method is probably the safest way to manage wounds in hard-times situations. Leave the wound open to allow the drainage of any pus resulting from infection unless you can close it safely. As long as a wound can drain, it should not lead to life-threatening infection, regardless of how icky it smells or looks.

Cover the wound with a clean dressing and hold it in place with a bandage. Change dressings daily to check for evidence of infection, including pain and tenderness, swelling, and redness around the wound, increased temperature, and pus in the wound or on the dressing. Plastic surgeons talk about a dressing style that is "clean and greasy" to minimize risk of infection and scarring while allowing a wound to heal. They use Vaseline gauze as the favored way of ensuring this. If needed, you can put a dollop of Vaseline on a piece of clean cloth or gauze, then wrap them in foil and sterilize them in you pressure cooker.

Home Instrument Sterilization TIP

STERILITY IS ONE HALLMARK OF MODERN HEALTH CARE, EVER SINCE JOSEPH LISTER (OF Listerine fame) and others developed the aseptic technique of surgery in the mid-1800s. With sterile supplies and techniques, surgery became much less likely to lead to infections that often were fatal.

You might not think you are doing surgery, but even things like wound care and other less advanced procedures benefit from sterility.

Sterile means an item has been treated in a manner such that all potentially infectious organisms like viruses and bacteria, plus their spores, found on the item have been killed. This also assumes the item is kept under sterile conditions until the time of use.

There are two basic ways we sterilize medical and surgical instruments nowadays: steam sterilization in an autoclave, or gas sterilization with Ethylene oxide.

You will notice that the classic boiling water or holding an item over a lighted match a la MacGyver are not among current techniques! Boiling water doesn't kill some spores, and the flame method can hurt the instruments or their user, so these are truly for use in extremis.

Ethylene oxide is highly toxic and thus dangerous, and is available only to instrument manufacturers and large hospitals. After gridcrash, for your group, the only practical method available will be sterilization by steam under pressure.

Autoclaves can be had on eBay, but generally are expensive: $700 or so for small used ones, although some made for tattoo artists and beauty salons are cheaper. An alternative to spending this much, as well as a dual use item, is an old-fashioned pressure cooker like home canners use. These alternatives usually are less than $100 brand new.

Sterilization must be done properly if it is to be effective. Clean and wash all instruments carefully to ensure they are free from body fluids and other debris before you sterilize. This is especially important if your instruments have been used before, but is important even when they are new. Use detergent and water, with copious rinsing (bleach is OK briefly but can pit or otherwise damage many stainless steels). Wear latex gloves if you have to handle contaminated items.

Pressure raises the effective temperature of the steam in the sterilization chamber so all pathogens are killed. The sterilization process is a function of both time and pressure.

Autoclaves reach higher temperatures and pressures than pressure cookers so they work faster. Pressure cookers need at least 30 minutes at 15 PSI and 250 degrees to be fully effective. Note that this is typically the highest pressure on most cookers and is DANGEROUS if not done correctly. Make sure your cooker is in good shape; replace worn items with approved parts. Follow manufacturer instructions and never let it run out of water. Once steam starts coming out of the pop-off valve, 30 minute at 15 PSI starts, so time this closely and remove the heat after half an hour. If there are any problems like loss of steam before that, turn it off!

Pressure cookers do not have a drying cycle, unlike autoclaves. You should package your instruments for later use after sterilization, and they must be dry before you package them. Ideally, you should seal

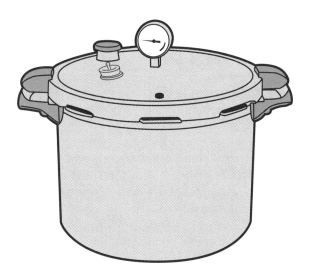

them first in autoclave bags, which conveniently are also easy to find on eBay.

If you don't have bags, or run out, you can sterilize a pair of forceps then use them to handle the items in the cooker for transfer to your patient care area at the time of use; the inside of the cooker will be a sterile holding area until you need them.

By the way: Pressure cookers should only be used for the sterilization of steel instruments. It is not for items that are heat sensitive, like latex gloves or liquids. Cloth drape sterilization is also not practical in pressure cookers due to their lack of a drying cycle.

You should be sure you have a pressure cooker of sufficient size to hold the largest instrument you wish to sterilize. This is also important because you will need to put a rack in the cooker such that the instruments are above the water and don't get wet during use; jars for canning can sit in the water, but instruments in bags should be in the steam only.

If a wound gapes open, you can bring the edges closer together with adhesive tape cut and rolled into the shape of a butterfly or dumbbell.

In survival situations, some degree of wound infection will be almost inevitable. To treat an infected wound, use this treatment daily until the signs of infection disappear:

Signs of Infection

- ■ Redness around wound
- ■ Increased pain and tenderness of wound
- ■ Warmth around wound
- ■ Swelling of wound
- ■ Discharge from wound

....

- ■ Place warm, moist compresses directly over the infected wound. Change the compress when it gets cool, keeping warm compresses on the wound for about 30 minutes three or four times per day to bring up the pus.
- ■ Drain the wound· by separating the edges and gently probing the wound with a blunt, sterile instrument.
- ■ Dress and bandage the wound.
- ■ Encourage the intake of a lot of fluids.

If you are without antibiotics and the wound becomes severely infected and does not heal, consider maggot therapy for cleaning (or *debridement*) of the wounds. Some maggots work better than others, as they will only eat dead tissues. These are the ones used by doctors (grown under sterile conditions to become certified "medical maggots").

- ■ Leave the wound open to flies for a day and then re-cover it.
- ■ Check it daily for maggots.
- ■ Once they develop, keep the wound covered but check it twice to three times daily.
- ■ Remove the maggots when they have cleaned out all the dead tissue but before they start eating healthy tissue. Increased pain and bright red bleeding from the wound suggest the maggots have reached healthy tissue.
- ■ Flush any remaining maggots from the wound repeatedly with sterile water or fresh urine.
- ■ Bandage the wound and treat it as any other wound; it should begin to heal normally.
- ■ Check the wound every four hours for several days to make sure all the maggots are gone.

Anxiety/insomnia. Teas made from mint leaves or passion flower leaves may help in reducing anxiety and allowing sleep, in some studies being shown to be as good as drugs in the valium class. Passion flower and St. John's Wort also may help with some drug addictions.

Depression. St John's Wort seems to be helpful for mild to moderate depression, as are omega-3 fatty acids. The latter also seem to be helpful in controlling some psychoses.

Rashes. In order to treat rashes effectively, you first need to determine cause. This may be difficult, even in the best circumstances. Dermatologists jokingly are said to use the following rules to treat rashes:

- If it is wet, dry it.
- If it is dry, wet it.
- Do not scratch it.

Use compresses of vinegar or tannic acid teas to dry weeping rashes. Moisten dry rashes by rubbing a small amount of grease or rendered animal fat on the area.

Remember to treat rashes as open wounds. Clean and dress them daily, watching for signs of infection.

Stings. Relieve the itch from insect bites and plant poisoning rashes by applying a poultice of jewelweed (*Impatiens biflora*) or witch hazel leaves (*Hamamelis virginiana*).

If you get stung by a bee, hornet or wasp, do not squeeze or grasp the stinger or venom sac, as this could force more venom into the wound. Instead, immediately remove the stinger and venom sac, if present, by scraping it out with your fingernail, a credit card or a knife blade. Wash the site thoroughly with soap and water to lessen the chance of infection. If you know or suspect that you are allergic to insect stings, always try to have an EpiPen or similar auto-injector with you.

Relieve the itching and discomfort caused by insect bites by applying:

- Cold compresses.
- Cooling pastes made of mud and ashes.
- Dandelion sap.

■ Crushed cloves of garlic or onion (use cautiously as these can cause skin irritation).
■ Coconut meat.

Animal Bites. These can be treated like other wounds, but are much more prone to infection, and thus more likely to get infected if closed with sutures. For this reason, make sure you clean them thoroughly by irrigation, removing any foreign bodies (like teeth) and dead skin.

Mammalian bites (remember that bats are mammals, too) carry the risk of rabies. If you can't get to a place offering rabies vaccination soon after a bite by any suspect animal, you have a few options. First, any bite should be *scrubbed* (not just rinsed or irrigated) thoroughly as noted above, but for rabies prevention, use a strong detergent. Studies in the 1950s seemed to show that benzalkonium chloride-based soaps help reduce the rate of rabies in bites if used within four hours.

Another possibility for these austere, desperate circumstances is (brace yourself) swabbing the wound within 4 hours of the bite with q-tip-like swabs soaked in nitric acid; both treatments obviously cause severe pain and lead to higher rates of tissue damage, infection and scarring. Still, you may need to avail yourself of these options, which will be better than what would otherwise almost certainly be a nasty death for the bite recipient.

If possible, observe the animal for 2 weeks. A rabid animal usually dies within 14 days, so if the perpetrator of the bite lives longer, it will be unlikely to have caused a rabies infection. Unfortunately, you may need to use an unpleasant preventive method prior to that.

Sprains and Strains. The accidental overstretching of tendons and ligaments (sprains) and muscles (strains) will cause pain, swelling, tenderness, and discoloration (bruised appearance). See *Fracture Care at the End of the World* for ideas on caring for fractures without the help of a doctor.

When treating sprains and strains, use RICE–

R — Rest the injured area.
I — Ice the area for 1-2 days, then apply moist heat after that.
C — Compress and/or splint the area to help stabilize and rest it
E — Elevate the affected area when possible

BROKEN BONES ARE PAINFUL, CAN LEAD TO LONG-TERM FUNCTIONAL LIMITATIONS, and if they are associated with major traumatic forces, can distract care-givers from less obvious but more life-threatening injuries. I teach my medical students and resident physicians an old aphorism: The worse the injury looks, the more you need to ignore it (as you look for other injuries and work to stabilize the patient).

Wait, you say: I have no X-ray machine! Well, you can use a stetho-scope for diagnosis of fractures in long bones. Simply find a bony prominence, where there is very little skin and muscle over the bones, on each side of the suspected fracture; these prominences are usually close to joints. Put a stethoscope over the bony prominence closest to the patient's heart, then tap on the prominence on the opposite side of the fracture. Listen to the character and intensity of the sound. Then, compare this to the sound produced when you do the same thing on the patients (uninjured if this is to work!) opposite limb. A difference is good at predicting the presence of a fracture. This trick is still used in some countries as either a cost-saving measure or due to lack of resources.

Many fractures simply cannot be treated ideally without more mod-ern tools than the *auscultation method* described above. Yet again, knowledge may help you make up for a lack of technology. In other cases, good first aid will make the patient more comfortable as you move them to more sophisticated care, and is useful by fostering heal-ing for the patient.

If you are in a situation where you don't have ready access to advanced orthopedic care, what can you do? For closed fractures (where the skin and other soft-tissues over the ends of the broken bone are not violated) you should immobilize the fracture. Use a splint designed for the purpose if available; if not, you can used rigid objects like wood, magazines and the like. Just make sure you pad these well, especially where the splint crosses joints and the site of the fracture. In very austere circumstances, you can use the patient themselves: Splint a fractured leg by binding it to the normal leg, or bind a broken upper extremity to the patient's torso.

Next, provide pain control. This is essential for patients whose limbs must be moved or straightened for rescue or transport. Most first aid and field care manuals counsel you to "splint them as you find them" but sometimes this does not work because of entrapment or other factors. One circumstance where "reduction" or getting the bones into a more normal position, is needed is with vascular compromise: Check the pulses beyond the fracture. If they are not there, you may need to pull the limb out to the correct length or otherwise manipulate it to ensure return of a pulse if you can't get them to a hospital quickly. Obviously, this hurts!

Once you have splinted or casted a limb, these pulse checks are essential: Swelling associated with the injury can compromise circulation, and if this happens, the splint or cast must be loosened to avoid long-term damage.

Remember non-pharmacologic techniques. Cold from ice helps control pain and swelling, as does elevation of an injured limb. Just make sure that the cold doesn't injure the underlying skin, and position patients gently.

For those with open fractures, commonly called "compound fractures," the major threat is infection. Any infectious material left in the wound is dangerous, as it will lead to localized infections like abscesses or osteomyelitis (a bone infection that could lead to failure of the bone to heal) or to widespread "sepsis" (blood poisoning). Because of this, unless you have access to sophisticated wound care techniques and very clean surroundings, you must not close the skin wound associated with the fracture.

From the outset, patients should receive pain control and have their wounds cleaned. Ideally, the patient will have made sure that they have current tetanus vaccination, making this dreaded complication, seen so often in WWI, unlikely. The early cleansing will help to reduce the risk of gas gangrene and tetanus.

Spanish Civil War surgeon Josep Trueta reported on the success of basic principles under the austere conditions in which he found himself—early casting of fractures, debridement, but no closure of the wound—in his 1940 *Treatment of War Wounds and Fractures*.

Trueta had worked extensively with industrial accident cases before the war, and applied his knowledge to the injuries he encountered during the war. Even though he was not an orthopedist, he wrote about orthopedic war surgery, and published a study on wound infections and mortality from wounds with recommendations for improved wound care.

After the Civil War, Trueta reported his experience as having only a 0.5% mortality rate and an 8% complication rate. In other words, 91% of his patients did well—an amazing reversal of the huge morbidity and mortality that previously resulted from open fractures.

Trueta's principles of wound management were: sterile technique during open debridement (removal of foreign matter, clotted blood and non-viable tissues) followed by plaster casting of extremity fractures to allow tissues to rest while healing.

Basically, the wound was cleaned extensively. After foreign bodies and dead tissues were removed, any bone fragments that looked too small or were stripped of their outer nutritive layer (the periosteum) were also removed. The wound was then extensively irrigated (using syringes to spray the irrigation fluid under pressure,) and the wound was left open once bleeding stopped. Next, a sterile gauze dressing was placed and the fractured limb was splinted in a plaster cast. As the wound healed, the plaster would literally soak up blood, plasma and pus that oozed from the wound. With time, the cast would need to be changed, as would the sterile dressing, but the fractures would heal and the rate of infection was very low, as described above.

NOTE

Although his book had the word "war" in its title, Trueta made a valid point: "Open fractures produced in road accidents or in industry do not differ essentially from those produced by aerial bombs or falling masonry." For that matter, farming and other sustainability activities have shown these types of injury as well.

Broken bones, especially compound fractures, often lead to death, amputation, poverty and other unpleasantness before the advent of modern medicine. During especially hard times you may need to have good basic fracture care in your skill set in order to get your patient to good care, or perhaps even to give that care yourself. Bone up on this information now!

Abscesses/boils. Apply warm compresses, which help bring the boil to a head. Then, you can open the boil through the head using a sterile knife, wire, needle, or similar item. Thoroughly irrigate out the pus using soap and water. Cover the site, checking frequently as you would with other wounds to ensure no further infection develops.

Back and neck pain. For pain in these areas that is unrelated to a fracture, you could try traction, using the weight of the body to stretch the painful area and diminish muscle spasms. For neck pain, you need a strap that cradles the chin and head; then, sit down with the cradle held from above and "sag" into the strap gently to produce traction.

For the low back, lie on a tilted surface, head down, with your ankles secured and your partial body weight providing the traction force.

In terms of austere drugs, clinical trials have suggested that daily doses of standardized Devil's Claw (*Harpagophytum Procumbens*) extract were better than placebo for short-term improvements in pain, and equivalent to 12.5 mg per day of rofecoxib (Vioxx). Trials looking at the effects of White Willow Bark (from *Salix Alba*) extract found evidence that daily doses were better than placebo for short-term improvements in pain, also equivalent to 12.5 mg per day of Vioxx. Finally, trials examining various topical preparations of Cayenne (*Capsicum Frutescens*) found moderate evidence that cayenne extracts applied over the painful area produced better results than placebo.

Emergency Childbirth. Women have been having babies outside the hospital with its intensive medical management of labor for millennia, and continue to do so in many other parts of the world to this day. It is reasonable to assume that every day women will have babies, and the little ones will continue to emerge regardless of the state of the world they enter. Because of this, it won't be useful to say "I don't know nothin' about birthin' no babies!" like in *Gone with the Wind*. Instead, families should become knowledgeable about childbirth and be prepared. After all: The "short trip" to the labor ward may not be so short. Many dads have had to deliver babies on the way in.

Under very austere circumstances, you may need to do your own version of the "get me some towels and boiling water" routine from the western movies of old. A thorough discussion of this topic is beyond the scope of this book. Suffice it to say that at the first signs of labor, get the best-qualified person available. Be calm, do not hurry or rush.

Learn the stages of labor, and how to assess them through simple bedside measures like timing length and frequency of contractions, feeling for the firmness of the contracting uterus and feeling for dilation and effacement of the cervix. Another trick is knowing when to slow labor to avoid tearing by allowing the perineum to stretch. Remember that you should NOT have to pull the baby or the placenta out. If you anticipate having to assist with emergency childbirth, have a delivery pack ready, but as always, learn: Try to learn about abnormal presentations, prolapsed and nuchal cords, performing episiotomies and repairing those as well as spontaneous perineal lacerations.

In the absence of the ability to perform Cesarean sections for complicated cases, though, we have to admit to ourselves that we might see the return of maternal and neonatal mortality levels not seen for over 100 years.

Finally: Remember that the baby will be a patient initially, and may need support for breathing and circulation. Try to have someone assigned whose sole charge is the care of the newborn.

Heart Attacks and Strokes: In the stressful times that may presage or result from the end of the world, we could expect to see more of these calamitous illnesses. Good CPR and defibrillation may fix some cardiac arrests, but some that could be saved now might not be in a darker future. Heart attacks and strokes both have the potential to benefit from aspirin, that simple drug, that can be improvised from bark as described in the fever section. Beyond that, supportive care with good attention to diet and activity with gradual rehab may be all we have to offer.

Major Trauma and Shock. These issues, like many of the upheavals of society predicating this book, are best treated with prevention. If someone should sustain major trauma from accident or from conflict, priorities will be simple things like making sure they can and do breath adequately, stopping the bleeding, and ensuring adequate circulation (the *ABC*s). Improvisation for these injuries will be difficult, but if you can provide enough advanced life support interventions you may buy a victim enough time to heal themselves, or to make it to a higher level of care.

In terms of breathing, make sure you know basic airway positioning maneuvers. Loss of consciousness can lead to loss of protective reflexes and muscle tone that keep a person's airway (from mouth/nose to the lungs) open. In the old days, we talked about "swallowing the tongue" to describe this. You could use safety pins through the tongue pinned to the lips to pull the tongue forward to prevent this in the deeply unconscious person.

You probably remember the story of the doctors on the flight who did a tracheostomy using a steak knife and the barrel of a ball-point pen, thereby saving the life of a fellow passenger. Nowadays, the knives are dull and/or plastic on commercial flights, but the principle still holds: You could use any sharp knife and a small hollow tube (like the barrel of a syringe) to do this procedure and provide a lifesaving airway. Here, more than perhaps any other subject, it is clear that knowing how to do something is as important as having the stuff at hand.

For supporting a person's breathing, you may not always want to do mouth-to-mouth, so it pays to have a mask or a resuscitator bag ("ambu bag"; look on eBay…) to provide artificial respiration.

Learning to stop external bleeding with pressure dressings, suturing and splinting will go a long way; most of the time you won't have access to major invasive surgeries, but being able to control external bleeding will help.

Finally, being able to replace lost fluids, either via the IV route or with oral or rectal fluid administration (see Tip) will help to reduce or prevent the circulatory shock, which with its loss of oxygen delivery to the tissues kills so many trauma victims after the so-called Golden Hour of trauma care.

Conclusion:
In most cases where you are caring for someone, calm reassurance and confident actions are helpful. Providing general "nursing" interventions like good hygiene, help with eating and positioning (turning the bed-bound patient frequently to avoid bed sores) and getting them gradually out of bed for rehab will go a long way as well.

For any of these treatments, you should try to keep some form of medical notes on each illness or injury you treat: what you thought was going on (based on observations you also record) and how you treated the patient, plus how they responded, in order to help future caregivers if more formal care should become available.

Any "end of the world" situation will call upon all of your skills, preparation, tenacity and ingenuity. While tenacity and ingenuity have been demonstrated many times to work, they may not always be there in the amounts you need them. I hope that you emphasize preparation and skill development in advance of a crisis. ●

CHAPTER 6

Ethics When There Is No Doctor

Ethics When There Is No Doctor

IN THE EVENT OF THE END OF THE WORLD AS WE KNOW IT, WE WILL BE FACED NOT ONLY WITH practical challenges such as obtaining food and providing health care, but also with philosophical or moral dilemmas. Any disaster will force us to confront changes to our familiar moral codes, and it pays to have thought about these challenges in advance, and ideally to have talked about them with others within your family or sustainability group. Finally, even though we do all these things to preserve life, we must recognize that all of us will die. The end of modern ease will be likely to change the way we die, so we need to be prepared for that, too.

An Ethic of Sustainability

SOME, LED BY BIOETHICISTS JESSICA PIERCE AND ANDREW JAMETON, STATE THAT WE ARE ethically bound to understand how to live in a sustainable fashion and that this includes not only our lifestyles (our diet and exercise choices, transportation modes, etc.) but also how we act as health care consumers. Consider, for example, that the developing world is burdened by 90% of the human disease today, but consumes only 10% of the world's health care resources.

Currently, health care is ecologically unsustainable: We know that since the 1970s, even before the oil embargo, people have recognized that health care generates prodigious volumes of disposable supplies used once and discarded as waste. We know about the energy intensive and technology driven health infrastructure. How can we reconcile these seemingly disparate demands?

Maybe you can find a "green health center" in your town or nearby that will be designed and run with an eye toward sustainability: less use of expendable supplies, eco-friendly design and services that focus on prevention and palliation, not cure-at-all-cost medicine. Such a health care team may even be interested in helping you and your group (family, friends or larger community) prepare for health in hard times by facilitating some of the steps described in this book.

On the other hand, maybe you can't stand all this sensitive save-the-Earth stuff and you just want to save your own skin, or those of your family and friends. You can be the most cynical person in the world, but you have to admit that there are clouds gathering and winds blowing that don't augur well for the future.

Maybe you take the third way: You see the benefits of both of these approaches. You want to live more sustainably with less deleterious impact on the world and your neighbors, but you also know you can't count on others to make the changes to get us off our current downward trajectory.

This discussion is obviously way too philosophical for one short chapter, and I will leave it to you to decide, but as I have been trying to hammer home for the entirety of this book, wishing does not make it so. YOU have to MAKE things happen.

Triage

AS WE TALK ABOUT HOW TO REBUILD A HEALTH CARE SYSTEM DURING AUSTERE TIMES, I THINK you need to make some other hard decisions first. Ethical considerations in the event of an epidemic of influenza, or other similar disaster or crisis, are going to be very difficult. Ideally, the criteria for making these decisions should be identified well in advance of their need. Consider that if you don't have these criteria in place, and all of a sudden are faced with the need to decide who will receive precious, limited resources such as ventilators, rationed medications or even food and water, you could find yourself confronted with a very difficult dilemma.

Picture a situation such as a sudden shortage of pain medications in your community, where a lot of people might have painful pre-existing conditions such as cancer. Deciding in advance how you will distribute or otherwise allot medications and reaching some agreement within your community on this will save you countless heartaches during hard times

You also need to decide how you feel dealing with other issues of triage of critical resources. Although these decisions have to be made regarding food, water shelter and other commodities, they may be most difficult to make when faced with people who are suffering because of injury or illness, who have severe pain or some other pressing need.

Another decision to think about is how you will deal with people who have unsalvageable injuries or untreatable illnesses. Some of these may have been pre-existing while others may occur after the crash. In either case, you may be confronted with having to make a decision to allow people in dire straights to die, providing only limited attempts to resuscitate or save them while offering them what comfort you can. Bear in mind that disaster has been defined by some as an event that overwhelms a community's ability to cope; your group will probably have to confront and cope with some of these situations.

As a physician, I believe it is generally a good idea for you to discuss end-of-life issues with loved ones. This is a difficult topic, but all too often we see families torn apart because they haven't come to these decisions in advance, and often argue about what course of action to take on behalf of a friend or family member. In the same vein, your group should discuss in advance how they will deal with these issues.

Security Concerns

ANOTHER TYPE OF TRIAGE CONSIDERATION IS THE SECURITY OF YOUR NEWLY CREATED HEALTH care group. Countless science fiction novels and movies have portrayed post-apocalyptic scenarios in which roving gangs of hoodlums, criminals or even cannibals have roamed around terrorizing those who were more prepared for the end of the world, as defined by the book or movie. Security, despite the somewhat hyperbolic treatment in these tomes, could be a concern during hard times.

Health care providers during the war in El Salvador, for example, and countless conflicts in other countries, plus personnel and clinical care sites of various nongovernmental organizations throughout the world, have faced these security concerns for a long time. In many cases, the belligerents have left them alone because they recognize that the clinics are neutral and provide service to all parties. In others, combatants have made the clinics and their staff targets when they have been suspected of sympathizing with one side or the other.

Perhaps the main difference between people who believe in sustainability and those with a more stereotypical survivalist mentality has to do with the issue of the use of weapons and other aggressive measures in hopes of ensuring security. As with other decisions discussed here, YOU must decide on which side of this line you, your family or your sustainable community will fall in making a decision about having and using weapons like guns.

The key comes in the recognition that conflict avoidance through negotiation and other measures are more likely to ensure your security unless you are willing to adapt a "shoot first, ask questions later" approach. We hope that infrastructure collapse won't leave us totally on our own, but must recognize that in some places and times, things have decayed to the point where security became an issue. In these circumstances, having a large group is one deterrent. Even if you are armed to the teeth, you will have to eat, sleep, bathe, eliminate waste and take a breather sometime. You can't be on guard 24/7/365. Even being "out in the middle of nowhere" is not a guarantee of safety.

Keep in mind the well-known aphorism that "if you live by the sword so shall you die by the sword". What I mean by this is that if you choose to engage in the use of firearms or other weapons for self-defense in one of the gridcrash scenarios envisioned in previous discussions here, you should recognize that you or those close to you may in turn be injured by firearms. You may choose to use other methods to preserve your security.

Having a Level I Trauma Center (serviced by paramedics, ambulances and rescue helicopters) is great now, but these services may be swamped or unavailable. Most physicians outside of a trauma center setting would have a great deal of difficulty, and not always a great deal of success, dealing with many knife and gunshot wounds.

I would suggest you look at other measures to help maximize your security. Here, you can learn a lot from hospitals in conflict areas that chose not to use aggressive means of defense.

Concealment is one method of security. Health workers during recent conflicts have hidden hospitals underground or in caves, traveled at night by side road or trail to avoid theft and harassment at roadblocks, and concealed the sick and injured in private residences rather than occupying fixed hospitals. See the *Guerilla Hospitals* tip for more details.

TIP | **Guerilla Hospitals**

SINCE THE BEGINNING OF THE ERA OF "TOTAL WAR" WITH WORLD WAR I, GUERILLA (or partisan) movements have fought asymmetrical campaigns against larger, more destructive state armies. Obviously, these movements have incurred casualties of their own, and in caring for them have had to develop clandestine "guerilla hospitals." The care they provided, and the innovations they fostered, have had an impact on the practice of medicine by the rest of the world, and in some cases provide lessons for us in our sustainability efforts.

.... ◀ **NOTE**

In most cases, guerilla hospitals were hidden, often underground, to avoid detection that may have provoked attack. Despite the need for isolation and frequent relocation in order to keep patients and staff protected, these hospitals had relatively low rates of infection. In large measure this was true because of meticulous attention to infection control procedures like we talked about in Chapter 4.

Labor in these hospitals was often provided by patients themselves: Those who were ambulatory worked within the limitations of their illnesses and injuries, helping to move other patients, to cook and clean, or to make needed supplies.

Lessons of improvisation and use of materials in imaginative ways can be seen in this setting, just like with POWs. The Viet Cong, for example, reportedly used out-of-date antibiotics discarded by the French colonizers. They also fashioned Instruments out of discarded items.

Lest one equate guerilla hospitals with backwardness, consider that in some cases, providers in these settings had forward thinking ideas and practices. Consider, for example, Josep Trueta, who worked for the Nationalists during the Spanish Civil War. His "closed method" for dealing with compound fractures caused by gunshot wounds was groundbreaking and reduced the amputation rate in not only that war, but after adoption by the British during World War II. He also did pioneering studies on the injury sustained by kidneys in victims of crush injuries, studies that impact today on the care of earthquake victims, among others.

Half a century later, and half a world away, Dr. Vo Hoang Le developed a novel approach to resource scarcity. As a surgeon working in the tunnels dug in the war zone by the Viet Cong, Vo utilized blood that patients had shed into their own chest or abdominal cavities, filtering it through gauze and transfusing it back into them on the operating table. This is one of the first modern instances of emergent autotransfusion, a technique practiced in trauma centers throughout the world today.

Remember the experience reported by those who opened their homes to people after Hurricane Katrina. If you don't want people to know about your preparations, including your health care prep, don't advertise. If you are forming a neighborhood alliance, you will have those around you "bought in" to your plan and will increase your security in this way, as long as tongues don't wag.

Other groups have used local health workers trained to be village medics, as described in the Village University section of this book. In keeping with the idea of concealment, villages in El Salvador routinely denied the existence of health workers in their communities; those who were identified were often arrested.

Simple, improvised and homemade local technology, plus natural herbal remedies, replaced supplies that were denied to the people by the belligerent parties.

Negotiation is nice if it helps you avoid conflict, but you need to have something that is of use to the other party in the negotiations, and must be certain that the other side is also willing and able to hold up their end of the deal. Beware those who have no powerful adversaries and nothing besides force to offer in negotiations!

Of course this discussion cannot occur without consideration of what to do when folks come begging: Can you turn away the sick or injured if you have the knowledge, skills and logistical wherewithal to care for them, even to a minimal degree, when the world around you is tumbling down? I would encourage you to consider, discuss and plan for these issues now, in the calm and security of our world as it is now. Your group will have enough on its mind when the world has changed, and engaging in philosophical discussions that are bound to generate controversy will take away time, energy and potentially trust when all of them will be needed most. Decide now if you want to have a clandestine hospital of your own, or when you might open it up to everyone.

Death and Dying During Very Hard Times

SOMEDAY YOU MAY BE CHARGED WITH CARING FOR A DYING PERSON, JUST AS THERE MIGHT come a time during which you will be called upon to meet all the needs of the living. Like so many of the skills we have neglected and shunted onto others, this is knowledge that was common to everyone only a few decades ago.

Indeed, we live in an era when kids (especially?) fear death in a way their Victorian playmates might have feared sensuality; those same playmates saw death as a part of life that was commonplace if not normal. Kids today know much more about how they come into being than how they will leave our mortal coil, in large measure because today, most of us in the West die in hospitals, often alone, in a highly medicalized passing.

It wasn't always so. Although the sick room of yore was used primarily to isolate and care for a potentially contagious family member, that was not its sole use. Those same rooms were also often a room for the last days of the dying. We can certainly envision a need during bad times for a similar dual-use of our sick rooms.

The end of the world would also mean an end to the prolongation of life regardless of patient suffering or societal cost, which many see as a good change. We all have a lot to learn about how to deal with futility in the face of illness, knowledge that fate may force us to gain when faced with the care of a dying loved one.

How you will face this situation emotionally is just as important as what you do, but what are the "non-clinical" interventions you can use to comfort the dying? First, remember the old aphorism that hope must not be allowed to die too soon before the patient. Being unable to cure does not relieve us of the obligation to care.

Do not do anything to induce or increase anxiety for the patient. Even though both caregiver and patient may know the truth, tradition holds that there may be some comfort in not letting it slip. On the other hand, realistic assessment of the situation, even when bleak, can be reassuring to many by providing them with room to develop feasible expectations and goals for the process. Control and closure are important characteristics that those with terminal illness repeatedly identify as crucial to a "good death." so don't deprive the dying person of these.

Confidence and support shown by the caregiver, even by keeping busy with small jobs in the sickroom, go a long way. Simply asking them how you can help is a comfort to many. Remember that most people fear dying much more than they fear death itself.

A major element contributing to this fear is the idea of being alone at the time of death: If possible, position the patient so they can see the activity going on around them. Keep the room well-lit, ideally with curtains to the outside world open. This is especially important because vision fades, which is distressing to the dying. Darkness only compounds this.

Conversely, hearing is felt to be the last sense to fail. A loved one stationed near the bed, quietly talking and comforting the dying person will provide them with pleasant final memories, and perhaps allow them to impart famous, or more crucially, meaningful, last words. Some also want a member of the clergy or other spiritual guide to be present at the end.

Although the movies typically show heroes complaining of being "so cold" at the time of their death, in reality we more often find that people in the process of dying complain of feeling hot instead. If the patient loosens clothing or removes covers, make sure he or she isn't too warm before you replace them.

Pain, either moderate or severe, is feared by the living, but surprisingly not always felt at the time of death; survivors of near death experiences have described it as bliss, peace and joy, freedom from discomfort and even "easy and pleasant." Ideally, though, if you have decided to stockpile medicine, you might want to keep some pain medicines and sedatives on hand for care of the dying, just in case. See the tip *Post-Crash Pain Control* for times when there is no pain medication available.

TIP ▶ **Post-Crash Pain Control**

PAIN IS PERHAPS ONE OF THE GREATEST OBSTACLES TO A HAPPY LIFE, AND EVEN possibly to a good death. Perhaps the greatest advance in history of medicine, and maybe even in the history of humanity, was the discovery and widespread availability of pain control medications. In the event of a failure of modern infrastructure, which now produces and provides the pain medications that so many people rely on, there are some fallbacks that will help minimize the pain, and more importantly suffering, of those patients with painful acute and chronic conditions.

Interventions that do not rely on drugs are called "nonpharmacologic" and in the realm of pain control comprise physical, behavioral and cognitive techniques.

Physical methods obviously are things like ice or heat application (that we frequently apply to ourselves after suffering sprains and strains.) Other physical modalities include massage and bodywork, acupuncture, and rest or immobilization as well as other positional interventions. Behavioral techniques include biofeedback, focusing on breathing and other relaxation techniques. Cognitive modalities include things like hypnosis, distraction/dissociation, guided visualizations and other imagery, and music. All of these techniques have been shown to be useful nonpharmacologic measures, especially in patients with cancer. While they haven't been shown by rigorous clinical trials to help, they have little risk and are helpful to most patients. Scientific theory for these tricks states that neurons along the pain pathways to the brain act as gates to slow or stop the transmission of pain impulses. These neurons are stimulated by some of the nonpharmacologic pain control techniques listed above.

Ever since Descartes, physicians, psychologists and philosophers have argued about this duality: mind and body in one person. For many physicians, this has manifested itself as a debate about pain and suffering. Physicians have noticed that people will vary from one to another, and even from time to time in the same person, in the amount of suffering they experience for a given amount of pain that they feel.

Many of our modern pain medications don't really block pain impulses; they just make you care less about the pain. Because of this, there has always been overlap between the pain relieving effects of medications and their psychological effects. Similarly, some of the plants we could use for pain control after gridcrash would work their effects by inducing psychological effects.

Ethnobotanical techniques, using native plants, MIGHT be one option for post-gridcrash pain control. Opium, from the opium poppy Papaver somniferum, is credited with being the impetus for the development of modern chemical pharmaceuticals: Purification of morphine in the early 19th century was a big step on the way to scientific medicine.

You might be able to find a way to grow opium, as seeds can be found for sale over the Net. So, you could "grow your own" although it might cause you all sorts of legal problems if governments find out. In the event of a world-wide catastrophe, though, you might get away with it. Once you have grown the poppies, you can harvest opium the old-fashioned way, by lancing the poppy pod and collecting the dry resin it exudes. If you are lucky, this would have about 1% morphine, plus some codeine and a few other chemicals (alkaloids, technically) as well. This could be taken orally or smoked for pain control. There are some older resources on the web from current licit growers and old botanical guides that you can find that might help in your attempt to cultivate the friend of Morpheus, the Greek god of dreams.

Another legally dicey way of providing pain relief would be our old friend dooby: THC in marijuana is reported by many to be a way they cope with pain and nausea. Again, you could run afoul of the law in choosing this method, and as in the case of poppy-based opium, you are using a natural product of suspect consistency and purity. Let the user beware.

The Institute of Medicine, in its 1999 report, "Marijuana and Medicine: Assessing the Science Base," stated that Scientific data indicate the potential therapeutic value of cannabinoid drugs, primarily THC, for pain relief, control of nausea and vomiting, and appetite stimulation; smoked marijuana, however, is a crude THC delivery system that also delivers harmful substances.

Research is still out on how best to utilize marijuana and its cannabinoid constituents in medicine, but again this is a widely available, readily cultivated option. Remember that the smoke from marijuana is probably as bad for your lungs as that from tobacco....

Finally, Salvia divinorum, more commonly called "Sage of the Seer" or "Magic Mint" is a weed that has become fashionable as a substitute for marijuana. It has been used for many years by indigenous peoples in Mexico, and currently is not illegal in the US. It has also been cultivated in the US and en masse in Switzerland. You can find vendors of the seeds for this plant online. As always, you assume all the risks when you go down this route.

Salvia contains a chemical called Salvinorin A that is presumably the main active compound; it is a potent hallucinogen similar in strength to LSD. It also seems to bind to opioid receptors and thus help reduce pain in mice, and it may have similar effects on humans as well. Unfortunately, you also buy yourself a ride on the crazy train if you use this drug for pain control, and its use for pain control is truly uncharted territory.

Hopefully all of this has convinced you of the need to get healthy before gridcrash, avoid injury and infection after hard times are here again, and to prepare by having knowledge and medicines on hand in advance.

Even after the pain is gone, thirst may persist. Keeping mucus membranes moist may help to reduce the "death rattle"—so distressing to the living—created by the motion of air over dry secretions in those close to death. Be aware of this and help keep your patient's mouth moist, even if they appear unconscious.

For most patients dying of "natural causes" like cancer or an infectious disease, unconsciousness supervenes, with about 2/3 being unconscious for the final six hours. Determination of death, which now relies on sophisticated monitoring devices like electrocardiography and brain scanning, will revert to older techniques. You can detect the absence of the pulse and heart sounds. You can also hold a glass under a person's nose or mouth and see if that fogs with their respirations. Finally, stroking eyelashes and seeing if that fails to elicit a blink reflex and checking pupils for failure to constrict on exposure to bright light will also aid in this determination.

Before determination of death is necessary, even though you may face futility in "curing" your patient, know that if you have freed them from loneliness and discomfort, and shown sympathy and love, you will have at least, at last, helped to heal them. ●

[CHAPTER 7]

Conclusion

LET'S RETURN TO THE SCENARIO FROM THE INTRODUCTION: THE CROWDED ER WITH ANGRY patients and the overwhelmed staff. Now, change the setting a bit. This time, we are in the US, England or any other western country used to a high standard of health care. Superimpose a few events on that country. The troubled banks, industries and economies worsen, unemployment soars, and on top of that, we now are in the midst or the aftermath of a bad flu season with resurgent swine flu. The work force absenteeism and social distancing measures from the flu have made the bad economic news even worse. The bad news feeds back on itself, and each setback in turn causes more worries. Oil prices, already on their way back up as of this writing, continue upward, driving up the cost of food, medicines and heating, all oil-dependent to some degree.

Whether you are a "survivalist" or a "sustainablist," your preparations (based in part on the information in this book) mean that the mishaps described in the introduction will affect you and your family, perhaps even your neighbors, much less than they affect the complacent among us.

Your need for emergency care, be it for a chronic illness, a pandemic disease or an acute injury, will be lessened because of your preparation and your hygiene and injury prevention efforts. You also know how to improvise medical

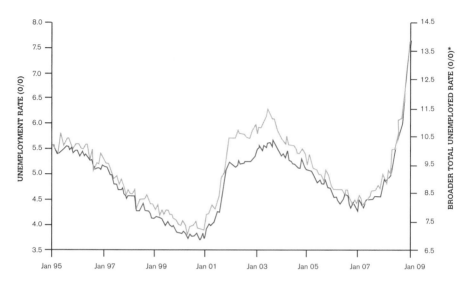

UNEMPLOYMENT RATE vs. BROADER TOTAL UNEMPLOYMENT*

*includes unemployed, plus discouraged workers, those working part time who want a full time position, plus marginally attached workers

care, make soap, minimize waste production and safely get rid of waste. You have stores of the medicines needed by those close to you, as well as other essential supplies. You may not have chosen to go so far as to educate a village doctor for your group, but things might not be that bad, and your simple efforts make so much difference already. You are able to help those near you who are in need as well, educating them where possible and bailing them out when the situation demands it.

Our world will change. If the past is to be our teacher, though, we need to admit to ourselves that change won't always be this ideal.

I began this project for a wide variety of reasons, but most importantly because I realized, after the birth of our first child, that my wife and I will create the world in which our children will live. For the next few years, they will be entirely dependent on us, and we don't want to let them down.

My wife and I hope that we can help create a safe, healthy, stable world for our kids, recognizing we don't totally control their fates. Thus it is that I also began this journey with the belief that we need to imbue our children with a sense of joy in being self-sufficient. We want them to be healthy, and also want them to be able to take care of themselves without having to rely on others for the basic things they need to live.

What can we do? Sustainable living seems to me our only choice: We live in an era when not only is the population of the world skyrocketing, but most of Earth's human inhabitants are demanding Western-style affluence: luxury, possessions and energy-intensive lifestyles. There is no proven way that will allow us to continue in this fashion. Rather, as parents we want to raise our kids with the values implicit in living more sustainably. This includes a lot of things, but sustainable health is probably the best overarching theme.

The other books in this series all echo this philosophy; if you want to blog or march or write letters to the editor or Congress in hopes of making things better, that is great, but you must also walk the walk. This work aims to help you live a healthy lifestyle, and to enable you to protect and restore health after hard times have come. Even if the presaged disasters don't come, you will be better off for having taken these steps. So will the world, if you use fewer resources and live a healthier life.

I wish I could tell you if we will face another Great Depression, or when oil will run out, or at what time on which day of the week solar flare activity will cause widespread power outages. The reality is nobody yet, not even Nostradamus, has been able to tell the future accurately!

What I can tell you is that the steps to mitigate the damage caused to our health by any of these events are simple. **What you know and what you can do count so much more than who you are or what you have.** We know what to do, and merely must do what we know. Not always so easy, then, but simple. I don't want my family, nor any other family, to face the dire straits envisioned in the scenario above, especially when avoiding it would be so simple.

We live in an age of unbridled prosperity that has led to unrivaled profligacy. Something, whether it be time and attrition or a calamitous event, will put an end to the life of ease which so many of us have taken for granted. My hope is that eventually, by beginning these efforts and sharing them with just a few people, we will create enough of a ground swell that each individual effort will coalesce into a larger, meaningful result for a planet and its people. ●

Survival Formulary:

MEDICINES FOR WHEN THERE IS NO DOCTOR

Medication (generic TRADE names)	Uses for drug
ANALGESICS	
NSAIDs	
ibuprofen MOTRIN (OTC)	Good general pain, fever controller
naproxen NAPROSYN (OTC)	Good general pain, fever controller
acetaminophen TYLENOL (OTC)	(variety of forms: liquid, tablet, rectal) Good general pain, fever controller
acetylsalicylic acid ASPIRIN (OTC)	(variety of forms: tablet, rectal) Above, plus heart disease and strokes
Non-Narcotic Analgesics	
tramadol ULTRAM	Less addictive than narcotics
OPHTHALMIC	
diclofenac sodium VOLTAREN *OR* **ketorolac 0.5%** ACULAR	Pain, itch control for the eyes
ANTI-INFECTIVES	
Systemic Antibiotics	
levofloxacin LEVAQUIN	Severe lung, kidney infections; also anthrax
amoxicillin/clavulanate AUGMENTIN	Head/neck infections; some GI bugs
doxycycline hyclate VIBRAMYCIN	Lung infections, most bioterrorism agents
clindamycin CLEOCIN	Dental, skin infections
metronidazole FLAGYL	GI bugs
sulfamethoxazole/trimethoprim SEPTRA (BACTRIM)	Mild urinary tract infections, staph
Skin Antibiotics	
silver sulfadiazine SILVADENE	Burns (not on the face)
polymyxin B/bacitracin POLYSPORIN (OTC)	Facial burns; infected skin wounds
Eye Antibiotics	
Erythromycin ILOTYCIN	Cheap, used for superficial scratches
polymyxin B/bacitracin POLYSPORIN	Cheap, used for superficial scratches

Medication (generic TRADE names)	Uses for drug

ANTI-INFLAMMATORIES AND ALLERGIES
Glucocorticoids

dexamethasone DECADRON *OR* **prednisone**	For bad allergies, rashes, asthma and croup

Antihistamines

hydroxyzine VISTARIL (ATARAX) (OTC)	For itch, anxiety and some nausea

CENTRAL NERVOUS SYSTEM

lorazepam ATIVAN	Stops most seizures; treats anxiety
haloperidol HALDOL	Strong sedative/antipsychotic

GASTROINTESTINAL
Antacids

calcium carbonate TUMS (OTC)	Good for heartburn

Anti-Diarrheals

loperamide IMODIUM (OTC)	Safe for most forms of diarrhea

Anti-Nausea

ondansetron ZOFRAN	Most causes of vomiting; few side effects

Proton Pump Inhibitor Antacids

omeprazole PRILOSEC (OTC)	Useful for reflux, heartburn

RECTAL STEROIDS/HEMORRHOIDS

hydrocortisone cream PROCTOCREAM-HC, anusol HC	Good for itch, swelling, pain

LOCAL ANESTHETICS:

1% LIDOCAINE injectable	Wound repair, fracture/dislocation care

NUTRITIONAL/SUPLEMENTS

prenatal vitamins w/folic acid PRENATE ELITE, others	General nutritional support for health

RESPIRATORY
Anaphylaxis Treatment Agents

epinephrine EPIPEN and EPIPEN JR.	For severe allergic reactions, shock

Asthma/Emphysema Combination Inhaler

ipratropium/albuterol COMBIVENT	For asthma, emphysema, bronchitis

Resources

CHAPTER 2

DIET AND NUTRITION GUIDELINES

www.health.gov/DietaryGuidelines/

www.nutrition.gov/nal_display/index.
php?info_center=11&tax_level=1

FIRST AID TRAINING SOURCE

www.redcross.org

www.icrc.org/eng

www.americanheart.org

onlineaha.org

MEDICAL SELF HELP GUIDE

www.fas.org/irp/doddir/milmed/family.
pdf

DISASTER RESPONSE TRAINING

www.ready.gov

training.fema.gov/IS/crslist.asp

CERT PROGRAM

www.citizencorps.gov/cert/

iTUNES UNIVERSITY COURSES

www.apple.com/itunes/whatson/
itunesu.html

WHERE THERE IS NO DOCTOR, ETC.

www.hesperian.org/publications_
download.php

LARGE COLLECTION OF RESOURCES

www.cd3wd.com/cd3wd_40/cd3wd/
index.htm

MILITARY MEDICINE TEXTBOOKS

www.bordeninstitute.army.mil/published.
html

SHIP'S MEDICINE CHEST GUIDE

www.fas.org/irp/doddir/milmed/ships.
pdf

MENTAL HEALTH FIRST AID MANUAL

www.mhfa.com.au/mhfa_manual.pdf

CHAPTER 3

FIRST AID KIT SUPPLIES VENDOR

www.adventuremedicalkits.com

www.remotemedical.com/Medical-
Rescue-Supplies

www.chinookmed.com

www.1staidsupplies.com/store.
php?crn=66

www.tasco-safety.com/first-aid-supply.
html

SICK/ISOLATION ROOM DESIGN TIPS

www.ready.gov/america/makeaplan/
stayingput.html

SPECIAL NEEDS PREP GUIDE

www.cdc.gov/family/specialneeds/

www.preparenow.org/pop.html

www.fema.gov/plan/prepare/
specialplans.shtm

www.nobodyleftbehind2.org

dept.lamar.edu/nursing/specialneeds/
final.pdf

CHAPTER 4

DEALING WITH DEAD BODIES

www.paho.org/English/dd/ped/
DeadBodiesBook.pdf

DISEASE MANAGEMENT GUIDE

www.health.gov/nhic/NewSrch.htm

DM GUIDE

www.impactbc.ca/
practicesupportprogram/
resourcesforclinicalpractices/cdm/
patientself-managementresources

www.rphworld.com/pharmacist/
viewlink-24165.html

Survival Supplies

ADVANCED DENTAL EMERGENCY KIT

- Gloves (sterile or non-sterile nitrile or latex)
- Faceshield or surgical masks and safety goggles
- 2 Dental Mirrors
- Explorer or Plastic pick/cleaner
- Explorer/probe double end # 5
- Dental Floss
- Baby Teething Gel
- Super Glue Gel
- Excavator, double-end # 38/ 39 or 38/40
- Plugger/filler, flat-bladed or double-end, # 1/2 or 1/3 or similar
- Elevator #301 or #304
- Extraction forceps # 150 and #151 universal upper
- Extraction forceps #150 and #151 universal lower (can use #75 as well)
- Zinc oxide-eugenol dental cement or Intermediate Restorative Material permanent filling
- Cavit temporary filling material
- Copalite cavity varnish
- Wax or glazed paper for mixing compounds
- Dry air dust cleaner for camera/camcorder (used to dry teeth before filling, etc.)
- Scalpel handle and #11 and #15 blades
- Needle driver, 4-5"
- Angle point tweezers
- Curved Iris Scissors
- Sutures: 4-0, 5-0, absorbable and non-absorbable, on Cuticular needle

- 25 gauge stainless wire (could use copper wire from core of power cords)
- Lidocaine 1% or 2%, with and without epinephrine
- Dental syringes and needles.
- Irrigation Syringe
- Cotton Balls
- Gauze 4x4s
- Alcohol wipes
- Salt and/or hydrogen peroxide for gargle/cleaning.
- Bleach wipes to disinfect instruments
- Battery-powered Headlamp (Petzl or similar)

LIMITED EMERGENCY SUPPLIES

Basic supplies needed for any type of sustainable community to reconstitute its own emergency health care system may include:

HAND HYGIENE
- Povidone/Iodine
- Scrub Brushes (could use dish brushes)
- Alcohol-based hand gels

PERSONAL PROTECTIVE EQUIPMENT
- Sterile Gloves- relevant sizes
- ExamGloves, Latex Free- relevant sizes
- Fluid Resistant Gowns
- Surgical and N95 Masks
- Goggles
- Shields
- Eye Wash Solution
- Hair Covers

INSTRUMENTS/EQUIPMENT
- BP Cuffs, Disposable
- BP Manometer
- Stethoscope
- Batteries-AA, AAA, D, C and device-specific
- Artificial Resuscitator Bags and masks, adult and child
- Pulse oximeter with heart-rate indicator (Nonin 9500, etc.)

- Tourniquet, one-handed model, like CAT
- Bandage Scissors or "trauma shears"

IV ACCESS/SUPPLIES
- IV Start Kits
- Micro Drip Tubing
- Adult Drip Tubing
- Blood Tubing
- Metri Set Tubing
- Syringes (2 or 3cc, 5 or10cc, 20 or 30cc and 60cc)
- TB Syringes or Insulin Syringes
- Injection Needles; 18Gx1½"; 20Gx1½"; 25Gx1½"
- Sharps Disposal Container (old glass jars with lids in a pinch)
- 20G IV Catheters
- 16G IV Catheter
- Winged "Butterfly" Infusion Sets 23GA &25GA

IV SOLUTIONS
- Lactated Ringers (LR)
- Normal Saline (NS)
- 5% Dextrose solutions
- In LR or NS
- In ½ NS
- In water
- Irrigation Solutions (could be home-made; see Tip)
- Normal Saline Irrigation Solution

RESPIRATORY SYSTEM SUPPLIES
- Nasopharyngeal and Oropharyngeal Airways
- Endotracheal tubes
- Oxygen Masks and Cannulas
- Suction Kits and Yankauer Suction Tips

ER/TRAUMA/SURGICAL SUPPLIES
- Scalpel handle and Blades- #10, #11, #15, #20
- Sutures
- General Instruments Tray
- Chest Drainage System and Chest Tubes- 8, 10, 12, 24, 32Fr

- Sterile Towels or Sheets
- Stainless Steel Basins, large and small (can be sterilized for irrigation, holding supplies, etc.)
- 2"X2" and 4"X4" Dressings;
- Adhesive IV Dressings (TegaDerm or OpSite, for example)
- 4" Gauze Bandage Rolls
- 1" Paper Tape
- Adhesive Bandages
- ABD Pads
- 3", 4" and 6" Elastic "ACE"-type Bandages
- Skin Staplers

GI SYSTEM SUPPLIES
- Nasogastric or Feeding Tubes, 8, 10, 12, 14Fr
- Catheter tip "Tumey" type syringes

GU SYSTEM SUPPLIES
- Urine Multi-Stix
- Foley Catheters

MUSCULOSKELETAL SUPPLIES
- Malleable aluminum splints (SAM splints; used for variety of splints)
- Plaster Impregnated Gauze Rolls 3" or 4"

OBSTETRICS SUPPLIES
- Delivery pack
- Catheter pack
- Cord clamps (3)
- Sterile and unsterile gloves (assortment of sizes)
- Sterile lubricant jelly
- Perineal pads, sterile 1 pack
- Dissecting scissors
- Kidney dish
- Sterile field
- Mayo scissors
- Disposable non-sterile gown/apron x 1
- Large plastic bags x 2
- Large biohazard bag x 1
- Baby bundle
- Towels (2)
- Baby blanket

- Hat & booties
- Disposable Thermal Wrap
- Disposable diapers

MISCELLANEOUS
- Sterile Lubricant
- Alcohol Wipes
- PVP Wipes
- Tongue Depressors
- Cotton-tipped applicators
- Garbage Can Liners/Bags
- Blood Glucose Testing Supplies
- Body Bags
- Safety Pins
- Povodine Iodine Swab Sticks
- Povodine Iodine Wipes
- Hydrogen Peroxide 3%

LINEN
- Disposable Sheets
- Disposable Pillows and Pillow Cases

PATIENT PERSONAL CARE SUPPLIES
- Facial Tissues
- Bedpans
- Urinals
- Diapers
- Pacifiers
- Cotton Balls

EXPENSIVE EQUIPMENT (Nice to have for intentional community, with trained personnel)
- Oxygen concentrator
- Portable ventilator
- Portable ultrasound machine (Sonosite, Siemens, etc.)
- Automated external defibrillator or monitor/defibrillator (Life-Pak, etc.)
- Femur traction splint

References

CHAPTER 1

Barrett, Kathleen: *The Collapse of the Soviet Union and the Eastern Bloc: Effects on Cuban Health Care.* Cuban Briefing Paper Number 2. Center for Latin American Studies, Georgetown University, Washington, DC 1993

Bednarz, Dan: "How Our Fossil Fuel Dependence Is Jeopardizing Our Health care System." *Orion Magazine.* July/August, 2007

Cook, Earl. "Some Health Aspects of High Energy Society," *Texas Reports on Biology and Medicine*, 33:25-44. 1975

Kline, A. Burt Jr. "Will Shortages of Raw Materials and Rising Prices Hurt Our Chances for Better Health Care?" *Public Health Reports* 90:3-9. 1975

McCarroll, James R. "Health costs of a reduced energy supply" *Environmental health perspectives.* 52:255-6. 1983

Santa Barbara, Joanna. "Foul weather ahead and we're low on gas." *Croatian Medical Journal* 47:665-8. 2006

Hanlon, P. and McCartney, G. "Peak oil: Will it be public health's greatest challenge?" *Public Health* 122:647-652. 2008

CHAPTER 2

Gardner E.J., et al. "Black tea--helpful or harmful? A review of the evidence" *European Journal of Clinical Nutrition* 61:3-18. 2007

Schneider, C. and Segre, T. "Green tea: potential health benefits" *American Family Physician* 79:591-4. 2009

Tattelman, E. "Health effects of garlic" *American Family Physician* 72:103-6 2005

White, B. "Ginger: an overview" *American Family Physician* 75:1689-91. 2007

Hughes, D.A., and Norton, R. Vitamin D and respiratory health. *Clin Exp Immunol.* 158:20-5. 2009

Clarke, J.O., and Mullin, G.E. A review of complementary and alternative approaches to immunomodulation. *Nutr Clin Pract.* 23:49-62. 2008

Lampe, J.W. Spicing up a vegetarian diet: chemopreventive effects of phytochemicals. *Am J Clin Nutr.* 78:579S-583S. 2003

Borchers A.T., et al. The immunobiology of mushrooms. *Exp Biol Med* (Maywood). 233:259-76. 2008

Lamas O., et al. Obesity and immunocompetence. *Eur J Clin Nutr.* 56:S42-5. 2002

Manz, Friedrich. "Hydration and Disease" *Journal of the American College of Nutrition* 26:535S-541S. 2007

Warburton, D.E.R. et al. "Health benefits of physical activity: the evidence" *Canadian Medical Association Journal* 174:801-809. 2006

Hasler G., et al. "The Association Between Short Sleep Duration and Obesity in Young Adults: A 13-Year Prospective Study" *Sleep* 27:661-666. 2004

Cohen, S. et al. "Sleep Habits and Susceptibility to the Common Cold" *Archives of Internal Medicine.* 169:62-67. 2009

Kalhoff, H. "Mild dehydration: a risk factor of broncho-pulmonary disorders?" *European Journal of Clinical Nutrition* 57:S81-S87. 2003

Szinnai, G. et al. "Effect of water deprivation on cognitive-motor performance in healthy men and women" *American Journal of Physiology Regulatory Integrative and Comparative Physiology* 289:R275-R280. 2005

Scully, D., et al. "Physical exercise and psychological well being: a critical review" *British Journal of Sports Medicine* 32:111-120. 1998

Everly, G.S., Jr. and Flynn, B.W. "Principles and practical procedures for acute psychological first aid training for personnel without mental health experience." *International Journal of Emergency Mental Health.* 8:93-100. 2006

Carson, Kevin: *The Right to Self-Treatment* downloaded at http://www.docstoc.com/docs/2986045/The-Right-to-Self-Treatment-Kevin-A-Carson-The-health 2 July, 2009

Mirhashemi, S., et al. "The 2003 Bam earthquake: overview of first aid and transport of victims." *Prehospital and Disaster Medicine* 22:513-6. 2007

Gilbert, M. "Bridging the gap: building local resilience and competencies in remote communities." *Prehospital and Disaster Medicine* 23:297-300 2008

Garakani, A. et al. "General disaster psychiatry" *Psychiatric Clinics of North America* 27:391-406 2004

Nardini, J.E. "Survival Factors in American Prisoners of War of the Japanese" *American Journal of Psychiatry* 109:241-248 1952

Husum, H. et al.. *Save Lives, Save Limbs* Third World Network, Penang, Malaysia. 2000.

CHAPTER 3

Smoak, B.L., and Petrucelli, B.P. "Medical Threat Assessment" from *Military Preventive Medicine: Mobilization and Deployment Volume 1* pp213-227 Downloaded at http://www.bordeninstitute.army.mil/published_volumes/mpmVol1/PM1ch11.pdf 2 July, 2009

Emergency Evacuation Planning For Special Needs Populations Inadequate Article Date: 24 Jul 2008

Downloaded at http://www.medicalnewstoday.com/articles/115919.php 2 July, 2009

Aldrich, N., and Benson, W.F. "Disaster preparedness and the chronic disease needs of vulnerable older adults." *Preventing Chronic Disease* 5:1-7. 2008 Downloaded at http://www.cdc.gov/pcd//issues/2008/jan/07_0135.htm 2 July, 2009

Welch, T.P. "Data-based selection of medical supplies for wilderness travel" *Wilderness and Environmental Medicine* 8:148-151. 1997

Boulware, D.R. "Travel medicine for the extreme traveler." *Diseases-a-Month* 52:309-25 2006

Callahan, M.V., and Hamer, D.H. "On the medical edge: preparation of expatriates, refugee and disaster relief workers, and Peace Corps volunteers" *Infectious Disease Clinics of North America* 19:85-101. 2005

CHAPTER 4

Coughlin, J.F., et al. "Old Age, New Technology, and Future Innovations in Disease Management and Home Health Care" *Home Health Care Management Practice* 18:196-207. 2006

World Alliance for Patient Safety: *WHO Guidelines on Hand Hygiene in Health Care: A Summary (Draft)* Downloaded at whqlibdoc.who.int/hq/2005/WHO_EIP_SPO_QPS_05.2.pdf 2 July, 2009

Drinka, P.J. "Report of an outbreak: nursing home

architecture and influenza-A attack rates." *Journal of the American Geriatrics Society* 44:910-3. 1996

Derrick, J.L. et al. "Predictive value of the user seal check in determining half-face respirator fit" *The Journal of Hospital Infection* 59:152-5. 2005

Boone, C.P., and Gerba, S.A. "The Occurrence of Influenza A virus on Household and Day Care Center Fomites" *Journal of Infection* 51:103-9. 2005

Escombe, A.R., et al. "Natural Ventilation for the Prevention of Airborne Contagion." *PLoS Medicine* 4(2): e68. 2007

Breese Hall, C. "The spread of influenza and other respiratory viruses: complexities and conjectures" *Clinical Infectious Diseases* 45:353-9. 2007

Weiss, M.M., et al. "Disrupting the transmission of influenza A: face masks and ultraviolet light as control measures." *American Journal of Public Health*. 97:S32-7. 2007

Jefferson, T., et al. "Physical interventions to interrupt or reduce the spread of respiratory viruses: systematic review" *BMJ* 336:77-80. 2008

Markel, H., et al. "Non-pharmaceutical interventions employed by major American cities during the 1918-19 influenza pandemic." *Transactions of the American Clinical and Climatological Association* 119:129-38; discussion 138-42. 2008

Hobday, R.A. "Sunlight therapy and solar architecture."

Medical History 41:455-472. 1997

Beggs, C. et al. "The ventilation of multiple-bed hospital wards: Review and analysis" American Journal of Infection Control, 36:250-259

Fabrice, C., et al. "Time lines of infection and disease in human influenza: a review of volunteer challenge studies." American Journal of Epidemiology 167:775-85. 2008

Brickner, P.W., et al. "The application of ultraviolet germicidal irradiation to control transmission of airborne disease: bioterrorism countermeasure." Public Health Reports. 118:99-114. 2003

Larson, E. "Hygiene of the skin: when is clean too clean?" Emerging Infectious Diseases 7:225-230. 2001

Katz, J.D. "Hand washing and hand disinfection: more than your mother taught you." Anesthesiology Clinics of North America. 22:457-71. 2004

Committee on the Development of Reusable Facemasks for Use During an Influenza Pandemic "Use and Reuse of Respiratory Protective Devices for Infuenza Control" (Chapter 3) from Reusability of Facemasks During an Influenza Pandemic: Facing the Flu The National Academies Press, Washington, D.C. 2006

CHAPTER 5

Paige, J.C. "The Importance of Understanding Human Misuse of Veterinary Medications" The Journal of Rural Health 18 (2):309-310. 2002

Brand, R. "Drugs Just a Click Away" State Legislatures 33:45, 47, 49. 2007

St. George, B.N. "Overseas-based online pharmacies: a source of supply for illicit drug users?" Medical Journal of Australia 180:118-119. 2004

De Guzman, G.C., et al. "A survey of the use of foreign-purchased medications in a border community emergency department patient population." The Journal of Emergency Medicine 33:213-21. 2007

Larson, Elaine L., and Grullon-Figueroa, L. "Availability of antibiotics without prescription in New York City" Journal of Urban Health 81:498-504. 2004

Hassel, L., and Arzuaga, P. "Importing prescription drugs: risky business" Employee Benefits Journal. 28:83-6. 2003

Erramouspe J., et al. "Veterinarian perception of the intentional misuse of veterinary medications in humans: a preliminary survey of Idaho-licensed practitioners." The Journal of Rural Health 18:311-8. 2002

Berlim, M., and Abeche, A. "Evolutionary approach to medicine." Southern Medical Journal, 94:26-32. 2001

Quaggin, A. "Prisoner and Doctor: Practice in a POW Camp" Canadian Family Physician. 28:1431-1432, 1434. 1982

Stallard, T.C. and Burns, B. "Emergency delivery and perimortem C-section." Emergency Medicine Clinics of North America. 21:679-93. 2003

Medicin Sans Frontiers: Normal Delivery and Usual Procedures for Various Problems from Obstetrics in remote settings (Chapter 4) - 2007, downloaded at http://www.refbooks.msf.org/msf_docs/en/Obstetrics/Obstetrics_en.pdf 2 July, 2009

Thorsness, L. Surviving Hell : a POW's Journey pg 47-51Encounter Books, New York, NY. 2008

Lam, G. "Medical Care in a Prisoner of War Camp" pg42-49 Downloaded at jsoupublic.socom.mil/.../jsom/JSOM_TOC_Binder-00-Spring08.pdf 2 July, 2009

Basic Survival Medicine. Environmental Information Division, Air Training Command Air , Maxwell Air Force Base, AL. 1981.

Dunlop, E.E. "Medical Experiences in Japanese Captivity" British Medical Journal 2(4474):481-486. 1946

Hoxha B., et al. "Field-improvised war surgery in Kosovo: use of kitchen utensils as surgical instruments." Military Medicine 173:529-33. 2008

Poidevin, L.O.S. "A Unique surgical experience in a WWII prisoner of war camp." Australian Defence Forces Health 6:4-8 2005

McKay, D.L. and Blumberg, J.B. "A review of the bioactivity and potential health benefits of peppermint tea (*Mentha piperita L.*)" *Phytotherapy Research* 20:619-33. 2006

Rosen, L.D., et al. "Complementary, Holistic, and Integrative Medicine: Colic" *Pediatrics in Review* 28:381-385. 2007

Werneke, U., et al. "Complementary medicines in psychiatry: Review of effectiveness and safety" *The British Journal of Psychiatry* 188:109-121 2006

Beran, G.W. "Disease and destiny-mystery and mastery." *Preventive Veterinary Medicine* 86(3-4):198-207. Epub Jul 17 2008

Roland C.G. "An underground medical school in the Warsaw ghetto, 1941-2." *Medical History* 33:399-419. 1989

"Disposing of Disposables" *American Medical News* September 28, 1970

Lewis, W.H., and Elvin-Lewis, M.P.F. *Medical Botany: Plants Affecting Human Health* John Wiley and Sons, Hoboken, NJ 2003

CHAPTER 6

Marco, C., and Schears, R.M. "Death, Dying, and Last Wishes" *Emergency Medicine Clinics of North America*, 24:969-987. 2006

Kompanje, E. "'Death rattle' after withdrawal of mechanical ventilation: Practical and ethical considerations" *Intensive and Critical Care Nursing*, 22:214-219. 2006

Parnia, S. et al. "Near death experiences, cognitive function and psychological outcomes of surviving cardiac arrest" *Resuscitation*, 74:215-221. 2007

"Symposium: The management of the dying." *Journal of the Royal College of General Practitioners*. 16: 59-67. 1968

Brentlinger, P.E. "Health sector response to security threats during the civil war in E1 Salvador." *BMJ* 313(7070):1470-4. 1996

Pierce, J. and Jameton, A. *The Ethics of Environmentally Responsible Health Care* Oxford University Press, New York, NY. 2003

Honey as Medicine?

Cooper, R.A., et al. "Antibacterial activity of honey against strains of Staphylococcus aureus from infected wounds" *Journal of the Royal Society of Medicine* 92:283-285. 1999

Zumla, A., and Lulat, A. "Honey–a remedy rediscovered" *Journal of the Royal Society of Medicine* 82:384-385. 1989

Haffejee, I.E., and Moosa, A. "Honey in the treatment of infantile gastroenteritis" *British Medical Journal (Clinical Research Edition)* 290:1866-1867. 1985

Moore, O.A., et al. "Systematic review of the use of honey as a wound dressing." *BMC Complementary and Alternative Medicine* 1: 2 2001 Downloaded at http://www.

biomedcentral.com/1472-6882/1/2 6 July, 2009

Ingle R, et al. "Wound healing with honey–a randomised controlled trial" *South African Medical Journal* 96(9):831-5. 2006

Paul, I.M., et al. "Effect of honey, dextromethorphan, and no treatment on nocturnal cough and sleep quality for coughing children and their parents" *Archives of Pediatrics & Adolescent Medicine* 161:1140-6. 2007

Barefoot Doctors and Medical Auxilliaries

Gong, Y.L., and Chao, L.M. "The role of barefoot doctors" *American Journal of Public Health* 72:59-61. 1982

Anonymous *The Training and Utilization of Feldshers in the USSR: Prepared by the Ministry of Health of the USSR for the World Health Organization* WHO Public Health Paper no. 56 World Health Organization, Geneva. 1974.

Zamiska, N. "Videos Teach China's Rural Doctors" *Wall Street Journal* Tuesday July 10, 2007 Downloaded at http://biz.yahoo.com/wallstreet/070710/sb118402239619261442_id.html?.v=2 2 July, 2009

"Life as a Village Doctor in Southwest China" Downloaded at http://www.nurseweek.com/features/dispatches/china/971024.html 2 July, 2009

Mullan, F., and Frehywot, S. "Non-physician clinicians in 47 sub-Saharan African countries" *The Lancet* 370:2158-2163. 2007

Cheap Models for Medical Procedure Training

Parwani, V., and Cone, D.C. "A novel inexpensive IV catheterization training model for paramedic students." *Prehospital and Disaster Medicine*. 10:515-7. 2006

Psychological First Aid

Everly, G.S., Jr., and Flynn, B.W. "Principles and practical procedures for acute psychological first aid training for personnel without mental health experience." *International Journal of Emergency Mental Health*. 8(2):93-100. 2006

Household Items for First Aid

Wendling, P. "Think Plastic Wrap as Wound Dressing for Thermal Burns" *ACEP News* August, 2008

Medication Shelf-Life

Lyon, R.C. et al. "Stability profiles of drug products extended beyond labeled expiration dates." *Journal of Pharmaceutical Sciences* 95:1549-60. 2006

Anonymous "Drugs past their expiration date" *Medical Letter on Drugs and Therapeutics* 44:93-4. 2002

Human Medicines that Are Safe for Dogs and Cats

Bren, L. and Sharkey, M. "Pain Drugs for Dogs: Be an Informed Pet Owner" *FDA Consumer Magazine* September-October, 2006

FDA Center for Veterinary Medicine "Treating Pain in Your Dog. Keeping Your Best Friend Active, Safe and Pain Free" Downloaded at http://www.fda.gov/downloads/AnimalVeterinary/ResourcesforYou/AnimalHealthLiteracy/UCM117773.pdf 2 July, 2009

Stop the Bleeding!

Doyle, G.S., and Taillac, P.P. "Tourniquets: a review of current use with proposals for expanded prehospital use." *Prehospital and Disaster Medicine* 12:241-56. 2008

Austere Dentistry

Anson, T. V. "The New Zealand Dental Corps as Prisoners of War" (Chapter 32), in *The New Zealand Dental Services* [part of: The Official History of New Zealand in the Second World War 1939-1945.] Historical Publications Branch, 1960, Wellington, N.Z.

downloaded at http://www.nzetc.org/tm/scholarly/tei-WH2Dent-c32.html 2 July, 2009

Johnson, C., and Geddes, D. "Remote Emergency Dentistry for Doctors" from *Oxford Handbook of Expedition and Wilderness Medicine* Johnson, C et al. eds. Oxford University Press, Oxford, UK. 2008

Austere Hormones

Banting, F. G., et al. "Pancreatic extracts in the treatment of diabetes mellitus: preliminary report. 1922." *Canadian Medical Association Journal* 145: 1281-1286. 1991

Strakosch, C, *The discovery of Insulin* Downloaded at www.historicgreenslopes.com/.../Booklet_The%20Discovery%20of%20Insulin%2006.pdf 2 July, 2009

Home Instrument Sterilization

Anonymous, "Sterilization: Microbiology" Downloaded at http://www.startlearningnow.com/articles/sterilization-(microbiology).htm 2 July, 2009

Fluid Administration without an IV

Grocott M.P., et al. "Resuscitation from hemorrhagic shock using rectally administered fluids in a wilderness environment." *Wilderness and Environmental Medicine* 16:209-11 2005

Expedient Wound Irrigation

Cyr, S.J., et al. "Treatment of field water with sodium hypochlorite for surgical irrigation. *Journal of Trauma, Injury, Infection and Critical Care* 57:231-5. 2004

Anglen, J.O. "Comparison of Soap and Antibiotic Solutions

for Irrigation of Lower-Limb Open Fracture Wounds. A Prospective, Randomized Study" *Journal of Bone and Joint Surgery, American Edition* 87:1415-1422. 2005

Fellows, J., and Crestodina, L. "Home-prepared saline: a safe, cost-effective alternative for wound cleansing in home care" *Journal of Wound, Ostomy and Continence Nursing* 33:606-9. 2006

Moscati, R.M., et al. "A Multicenter Comparison of Tap Water versus Sterile Saline for Wound Irrigation" *Academic Emergency Medicine* 14: 404-409 2007

Fracture Care at the End of the World

Lippmann, R.K. "The Use of Auscultatory Percussion for the Examination of Fractures" *Journal of Bone and Joint Surgery, American Edition* 14:118-126. 1932

McLachlin, A.D. "Treatment of Fractures in Mass Casualties" *Canadian Medical Association Journal* 67:530-532. 1952

Guerilla Hospitals

Cu Chi Tunnels, Downloaded at http://www.mazalien.com/the-cu-chi-tunnels.html 2 July, 2009

Trueta, J. "The Treatment of War Fractures by the Closed Method" *Proceedings of the Royal Society of Medicine* 33:65-74 1939

Post-Crash Pain Control

Menefee, L.A., and Monti, D.A. "Nonpharmacologic and Complementary Approaches to Cancer Pain Management" *Journal of the American Osteopathic Association* 105: S15-20. 2005

Freemantle, M. "Morphine" Downloaded at http://pubs.acs.org/cen/coverstory/83/8325/8325morphine.html 2 July, 2009

Mika, E.S. "Studies on the Growth and Development and Morphine Content of Opium Poppy" *Botanical Gazette* 116:323-339 1955

Sheffler D.J., and Roth, B.L. "Salvinorin A: the "magic mint" hallucinogen finds a molecular target in the kappa opioid receptor." *Trends in Pharmacologic Sciences* 24:107-9 2003

Joy, J.E., et al, eds. *Marijuana and Medicine: Assessing the Science Base* National Academy Press, Washington, D.C. 1999

Index